3 6014 00066 3533

DATE DUE

7/16/14			
AUG 08 2014			
SEP 08 2014			
NOV 05 2014			

PRINTED IN U.S.A.

2/14 636.7 RID $16-

REED MEMORIAL LIBRARY
1733 Route 6
Carmel, NY 10512
845-225-2439
www.carmellibrary.org

How to Treat Your Dogs and Cats with Over-the-Counter Drugs

Robert L. Ridgway, DVM

Dr. Ridgway is the author of eighteen professional journal articles and five professional auto tutorials.

REED MEMORIAL LIBRARY
1733 Route 6
Carmel, NY 10512
845-225-2439
www.carmellibrary.org

iUniverse, Inc.
Bloomington

How to Treat Your Dogs and Cats with Over-the-Counter Drugs

Copyright © 2011 Robert L. Ridgway, DVM

All rights reserved. No part of this book may be used or reproduced by any means, graphic, electronic, or mechanical, including photocopying, recording, taping or by any information storage retrieval system without the written permission of the publisher except in the case of brief quotations embodied in critical articles and reviews.

The information, ideas, and suggestions in this book are not intended as a substitute for professional medical advice. Before following any suggestions contained in this book, you should consult your personal veterinarian. Neither the author nor the publisher shall be liable or responsible for any loss or damage allegedly arising as a consequence of your use or application of any information or suggestions in this book.

iUniverse books may be ordered through booksellers or by contacting:

iUniverse
1663 Liberty Drive
Bloomington, IN 47403
www.iuniverse.com
1-800-Authors (1-800-288-4677)

Because of the dynamic nature of the Internet, any web addresses or links contained in this book may have changed since publication and may no longer be valid. The views expressed in this work are solely those of the author and do not necessarily reflect the views of the publisher, and the publisher hereby disclaims any responsibility for them.

Any people depicted in stock imagery provided by Thinkstock are models, and such images are being used for illustrative purposes only.

Certain stock imagery © Thinkstock.

ISBN: 978-1-4502-9005-0 (pbk)
ISBN: 978-1-4502-9007-4 (clth)
ISBN: 978-1-4502-9006-7 (ebk)

Printed in the United States of America

iUniverse rev. date: 06/20/2011

To my wife, Carolyn, my daughter, Joan, and my son-in-law, Rob

Contents

Foreword xiii
Preface xv

CHAPTER 1
Trauma, Seizures, and Disease Prevention 1

Cleaning Ears 1
Complications in Delivery of Pups and Kittens 2
Coughing 2
Dogs Fetching Balls 3
Eyes 5
Fat Dogs and Cats (Obesity) 6
Embedded Collars 6
Immunizations 7
Immunization Reactions 7
Impacted Anal Glands or Scooting the Rear End on the Floor 8
Lameness 8
Self-Trauma and Self-Mutilation 9
Seizures 10
Toenails Trimmed and Bleeding 11
What Food Should I Feed? 11

Chapter 2:
Behavioral Problems 13

   Messing in the House or Defecating on Floors 13
   Petting-Induced Aggression in Cats 14
   Urine Spraying in Cats... 14
   Skunk-Sprayed Dog or Cat 15
   Feces-Eating (Coprophagy) 16

Chapter 3:
Intestinal Disorders 19

   Bad Breath (Halitosis) 19
   Constipation 20
   Passing Intestinal Gas (Flatulence) 20
   Hairballs 21
   Loose Stools 22
   Meat-Exclusive Diets 25
   Motion Sickness Or Traveling with Pets 26
   Intestinal Parasites 29
   Vomiting 34

Chapter 4:
Skin Conditions 35

   Allergic Response to Plastic Feeding Bowls 35
   Barbering: Excessive Grooming of Cats 36
   Biting Flies 36
   Demodex Red Mange Hair Loss 37
   Dull Hair Coat 38
   Fleas 39

Fly Strike 40

Hair Loss: Fleas and Demodex 41

Hot Spots 42

External Parasites: Ear Mites, Scabies, Lice 43

Ringworm Fungal Infections 46

Sebaceous Gland Cysts 47

Skin Wounds 48

Chapter 5:
The Eyes Have It 49

Cherry Eye 49

Bulging or Proptosis Out of the Eye Socket 50

Eye and Nasal Discharge in Cats 51

Foreign Body behind the Third Eyelid 51

Inward Rolling of the Eyelid Margin (Entropion) 52

What to Do with Hair in the Eyes of Dogs and Cats 53

Eye Infections 54

A Single Ruptured Blood Vessel on the White of
the Eye (Sclera) 54

Chapter 6:
Skin Challenges to be Conquered 56

Sores around the Ears of Cats 56

Miliary Dermatitis of Cats or Feels like Fine Sand
on the Skin 57

Mosquito Bite Hypersensitivity in Cats 57

Excessive Hair Shedding of Dogs 58

Hair Loss between the Eyes and Ears of Cats 58

Hunting Season and Working Dog Foot Pad Trauma..... 59
Lack of Pigment on the Nose or Nasal Vitiligo 60
What Shampoo Should I Use? 60
My Dog Has Dry Skin. What Can I Do? 60

CHAPTER 7:
Easy to Prevent, but often Hard and Expensive to Treat..... 62

Rocky Mountain Spotted Fever 63
Salmon Poisoning (Pacific Northwest) 63
Antifreeze in Cabin Toilets in Mountain or Ski Areas..... 64
Grape or Raisin Toxicity 65
Feeding Raw Eggs 65
Chocolate Poisoning 66
Treatment: 66
Lyme Disease 66
Problems with Homemade Cat Foods 67
Tick Paralysis 68
Plants in and around the House that are Poisonous
to Pets 69
Poison Help Centers 70
Household Hazards 71
Rabies 73
Distemper 74

CHAPTER 8:
Nutrition and Other Digestive Tract Occurrences 75

My Pet is not Eating. What Should I do? 75
Should I Feed Table Scraps to My Pet? 76

Feeding Omega-3 Fatty Acids 76
Yellow Tooth Syndrome 77
Aging Cats and Dogs by their Teeth 78
Vocal Cords Blocking the Wind Pipe (Trachea) 80
The Danger of Sewing Needles 80
Sewing Thread—a Deadly Hazard for Cats 81
A Special Note about Tapeworms 81
Using Panacur for Treatment of Hookworms,
Roundworms, Whipworms, and Tapeworms 82
Coccidia Treatment with Marquis (Ponazuril) 85

CHAPTER 9:
Trauma and Other Uh-Oh Occurrences 87

Sunstroke or Excessive Body Temperature 87
Lip Swelling Due to Angioneurotic Edema or
Angioedema of Dogs 89
Hospitalization Due to Dog Bites 89
Mumps 90
Rattlesnake Bites 91
Lying to Your Veterinarian 92
Foreign Bodies in the Nose 92
Reverse Sneeze 93
Kennel Cough 93
Grass Awns 94
Umbilical Hernias 95
Head Tilt 95
Pets and Yards Recently Sprayed with Chemicals 96
Ear Medicine Causing Hypersensitivity to Drugs 96

Ruptured Intervertebral Discs 97
Gunpowder and Dogs 98
Separation Anxiety of Dogs 98
Open Draining Sore Under the Eye 99

About the Author 101
Index 103

Foreword

When I first heard that well-known veterinarian, Bob Ridgway, was writing a book regarding problems that ordinary people like you and I have with our pets and what we can do to help them, I got really excited! Although I am a physician, my knowledge of veterinary medicine is very limited. Oh, sure, I know that certain foods, such as chocolate and grapes are very dangerous for pets. I was aware that certain medicines for humans are toxic to dogs. What I didn't know before I read this book was the correct dosages, dosing intervals, and duration of treatment for the medicine that can be used to treat pets. This book outlines in clear and easily understandable recommendations the proper dosing of available medicines. That's exactly what you and I need to know to avoid overdosing our pets!

I would like to tell you something about the author. Dr. Ridgway graduated from Kansas State University College of Veterinary Medicine. Thereafter, he took a small-animal internal medicine residency at the University of California at Davis. He is board certified in veterinary preventative medicine and also in laboratory animal medicine. He served as a lieutenant colonel in the US Army, where he was on the team that acquired military working dogs, often traveling to Germany for this purpose. Since leaving the army, he has been a practicing veterinarian in Orlando, Florida. He does between four hundred fifty and five hundred surgical procedures per month. He is an authority on the subjects covered in his book.

This book is the only authoritative guide that I am aware of that outlines in detail the proper use of over-the-counter drugs to treat your pet. Importantly, the book alerts the reader to conditions that required prompt attention by a veterinarian rather than attempting to treat the conditions at home. Thus, it is an excellent guide to a pet owner as to when he or she should not treat his or her pet. This is just as important as knowing when to treat without consulting a veterinarian.

With this book as guide, the reader will better be able to discern what he or she can do for his or her pet using over-the-counter medications. It thus allows the pet owner to recognize and treat many conditions yet prevents over-treating and overdosing his or her pet. To me, this is invaluable information. Therefore, I will keep this valuable resource in my collection of reference books. It will help me be a better pet owner. I believe the book will do the same for you! It's not meant to replace a timely visit to the veterinarian, but it certainly is an excellent guide for everyday use. It fills a void, and the author is to be commended for bringing us a wealth of useful information. I look forward to reading future editions of this fine reference.

Charles H. Beckmann MD, FACP, FACC, FAHA
Professor of Medicine, ret.
Uniformed Services University of the Health Sciences
Bethesda, Maryland & San Antonio, Texas

Preface

This book contains descriptions of medical conditions and over-the-counter treatments for diseases such as hookworms, bad breath, loose stools, red mange (Demodex mange), heartworm, scabies, choking, skunk spray, impacted anal glands, fleas, and many others that are found in dogs and cats that can be treated with over-the-counter drugs. This book is a result of my many years as a veterinarian and being asked many questions, such as, "How can I?" "Where can I?" and "Is there something I can do?"

The majority of pet health issues are due to owner neglect. This book is designed to teach owners the art of preventive medicine in their own homes. During my years practicing veterinary medicine, I have noted that folks are desperate to help their dogs or cats but do not have the financial means or inclination to provide for a trip to see a veterinarian. Furthermore, many have attempted to treat their dogs or cats with over-the-counter medication but have had no clue as to the dose, frequency, or number of treatments necessary to heal the condition. Unfortunately, some have thought that if a little over-the-counter drug is good, then a bunch more should be even better. This is a *big* mistake. Overdosing has resulted in many a dog or cat being treated for toxicity—or even being killed—as a result of its owner's attempts to aid it.

This book recognizes that your ability to diagnose a condition may, in fact, be in "the twilight zone." However, you certainly can recognize hair loss, pale gums, loose stools, poor breath, and perhaps may have even seen those lovely critters called worms coming from your dog or cat. This book will aid you by providing descriptions of the conditions and possible over-the-counter medications that will hopefully resolve the condition you recognize as needing to be treated. This is not a first-aid book; if the condition cannot be treated with an over-the-counter drug or home remedy, it is not included. I have violated this rule a few times because I have received so many questions about some condition. I have mentioned them, but have indicated that—in my professional judgment—you cannot adequately diagnose and treat the condition safely or there are no over-the-counter medications that will treat the condition.

I am excited that you have purchased this book, and I look forward to hearing how you were able to overcome the health conditions in your pet. The main issue you will have is deciding what your pet has in order to properly treat the condition. Sometimes the obvious is not so obvious, and your experience in deciding what disease process is present may not be quite up to par. However, even if you happen to mistreat your pet with any medication in this book with the indicated dosages within this book, then there should not be any real issues—other than the condition you treat may not improve. You certainly always have the best option available to you and that is to take your pet to see your favorite veterinarian; he or she will be most happy to assist you with your pet's health issues. We strongly recommend that you take your pet to see the veterinarian.

Obviously, your use of the enclosed information is your own voluntary decision on the behalf of your pet. If you happen to be wrong and cause injury to your pet due to a misdiagnosis of the condition, an overdose with over-the-counter medicine, or any other type of improper treatment, neither the publishing company nor the author bears any responsibility for your decisions or actions.

We hope that this book will help to aid in better decision-making, dosing, and proper medication selection by you. The book provides guidelines only; no one but you is involved in the decision-making process of what you do for your pet. Alas, you stand alone.

Here is to the health of your pet and to you for taking great care for your pet.

As the book was written, many suggestions for inclusions were provided to the author. It is my desire to follow-up on issues with more conditions and treatments. Since it is impossible to come up with all the issues that dog or cat owners have or need over-the-counter help for, we need your help for future editions. An opportunity is provided for you to provide comments, suggestions, and inquires by writing to the following address: Dr. Bob, PO Box 690164, Orlando, FL 32869-0164. If we get tons of responses, it will be impossible to respond to your individual correspondence. However, ideally you can find your answer in the next book. For those who are computer whizzes, you can e-mail: dogcatotc@gmail.com.

Chapter 1

Trauma, Seizures, and Disease Prevention

I do not give a damn for a man that can only spell a word one way.
—*Mark Twain*

In this chapter you will learn to recognize a variety of issues in dogs and cats that, with good care and observation, will allow you to avoid further health issues, prevent trauma, maintain your pet's health, and diminish or prevent unhealthy conditions. Sometimes what appears to be is not reality, but with knowledge, you are more apt to be aware and recognize issues more quickly.

Cleaning Ears

Many pets have dirty ears or dirty ears with ear mites, leading to terrible ear infections that one would not even imagine could possibly become so bad. It is a good idea for you to look into your pet's ears. Dogs with long, floppy ears are much more prone to ear infections compared to breeds that have ears that stand up.

Treatment:

You will need mineral oil and warm water. Fill one ear with mineral oil and massage vigorously and then do the same to the other ear.

Allow head shaking after each massage. Repeat this process three times for each ear. Then fill an ear with warm water and massage vigorously. Do the same thing to the opposite ear and repeat this process two times. Normally, this short process will clean the ears quite well. It is difficult to see deep into the ears of dogs and cats, but I think you will be pleased by this procedure. If you feel that your pet needs a second round, do it. It will not hurt the pet. This procedure is somewhat messy—oil can soil couches or other furniture—so be aware.

Complications in Delivery of Pups and Kittens

The biggest problem I have noted when a pregnant dog or cat tries to deliver her young is that the family makes a three-ring circus out of the event and everyone tries to get in on the act. The result is that the dog or cat will not deliver. I have had many come to me, but I have only done one Caesarian delivery. All I have done is put the animal into a cage, put a towel over the cage, turn out the lights, and leave it alone. The animals have always delivered without any problems. The pet did not deliver at home because of all the attention that was given—all the dog or cat wanted was seclusion and quiet. The mama-to-be would prefer to have her young in private.

Treatment:

Put your mama-to-be in a room, get everyone out of the room, and turn out the lights. After an hour, check on her. Normally, she will have had the young. If it goes beyond two hours, take her to your veterinarian.

Coughing

Coughing is very common in dogs and cats. However, there are so many difficult causes that are dangerous to your pet's health—including heart failure or congestive heart failure—that I cannot recommend a safe treatment without a professional diagnosis. However, you can certainly feel comfortable with the diagnosis of your pet's doctor. I recommended that you take your pet to see the most illustrious and honorable doctor of veterinary medicine. However, if your pet's coughing keeps you awake at night, you can use the following palliative medicine to help reduce the cough. Reducing your pet's cough will allow you to get some sleep.

Palliative Treatment:

Robitussin DM can be obtained and given. For small animals, give 2 cc or ½ teaspoon. For large dogs, give 5 cc or 1 teaspoon. This usually will reduce the amount of coughing at night.

Dogs Fetching Balls

When we play with our dogs, we often throw an object, such as a ball, that the dog will retrieve and return to the owner. A small ball might get caught in the dog's throat. If you have to take the dog to the doctor, it will be too late since the dog will die of asphyxiation before you can get there. First, you should make sure that the ball is too large to get stuck in the dog's throat. Second, you must treat this condition on the spot because later is too late for your pet.

Treatment:

Follow these simple steps to dislodge the object from the dog's throat or mouth:

- Give your dog a shake to try to dislodge the obstruction.
- You may have to put your finger into its mouth to try to dislodge it.
- If the object is too far back to retrieve, be careful not to push it further into the throat or mouth.
- Large dogs will need to have the back legs lifted off the ground before shaking the body. If the dog is small, lift up the dog's back end, making sure that the rear end is higher than the head, or lift the dog and shake with the head down to try to dislodge the ball or object.

If unsuccessful, use a Heimlich maneuver as soon as possible:

- Put your arms under the dog's belly and feel the last rib with your thumb.
- Make a fist, place your other hand on your fist, and give a quick jerk or push upward to force air out of the lungs to expel the item from the throat. Enough force should be applied that the body of the dog comes off the ground or floor as you move your arms into its belly.
- It may be necessary to repeat the maneuver three or four times. If nothing comes out, there is one last resort.

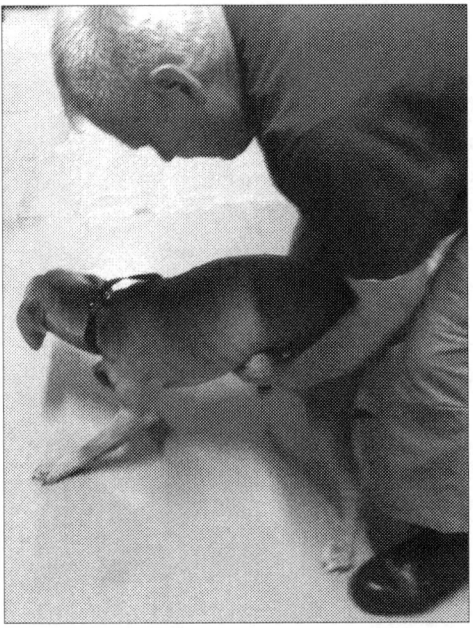

Figure 1: Performing the Heimlich Maneuver

Place the dog flat on the ground on either side and slap its chest really hard. If necessary, repeat three or four times. Unfortunately, if this does not work, it will be impossible to get to a veterinary hospital with the dog alive. In this do-or-die situation, you must get the object out. You will have about four minutes or less to complete the procedure. If not successful with the above two methods, you can—as a last desperate resort—perform a tracheotomy. To do a tracheotomy, you must have a knife to cut through the skin to the trachea. Since the trachea is rather close to the skin, it is important to keep your cool and not panic and slit the throat. Visualize the trachea and then poke a hole between the two tracheal rings. Place the barrel of a ballpoint pen into the hole so that the dog can breathe through the pen barrel. Take the dog to your veterinarian and let them do the surgery to repair your handiwork.

Eyes

Your pet's eyes are so important and so easy to destroy that we will focus on the one area that you can help your pet. Anything other than what we discuss here should be examined by a doctor of veterinary medicine. Your pet only has two eyes—don't let them be destroyed. They can look good today and be gone tomorrow. First, we will discuss dry eyes. If your pet's eyes are not shiny, look dry, and have gunk accumulating on the eye and eyelids, then obviously the dog has dry eyes. One would think that folks would clean and provide moisture to the eyes, but you would be surprised at how many dry eyes I see with no effort whatsoever to aid the poor critter. Cleaning the area around the eyes and the eyelids and applying artificial tears would work wonders for your poor pet's eyes.

Treatment:

OTC medicines—artificial tears—for dry eye are available at pharmacies and some grocery stores and Walmart. There are very watery (low-viscosity) artificial tears and very thick (high-viscosity) artificial liquid tears. Since the thicker tears tend to hang around on the eyes longer, put the thick drops on the eyes as frequently as possible. The minimum is four times per day. My personal favorite is ointment because it will remain in the eye longer than a liquid. Your pet will thank you for your efforts. A good ointment is GenTeal ophthalmic ointment; it is available at pharmacies and tends to stay in the eye longer, which is better for dry eyes.

Fat Dogs and Cats (Obesity)

Obesity in dogs and cats is a really bad condition that can lead to many other health conditions, including diabetes. Obesity is a very common issue for pets; to overcome it, you must be willing to work with the diet and the pet. Without your commitment to help the animal reduce weight, it is a lost cause. Many people mistakenly think that dogs and cats need three meals per day. Your veterinarian can prescribe medications; however, if you have the commitment to reduce your pet's weight, you can do it easily. All it takes is calorie reduction and bit of time.

Treatment:

All you need to do is to cut the amount of food you feed. If you feel that you need to feed twice per day, cut the morning ration in half and feed one half in the morning and the other half in the evening. If you cannot handle that, there are diets to reduce the weight of dogs and cats that can be purchased at pet stores.

Embedded Collars

This is a sad, sad condition to treat. I have had some wounds so deep into the tissue that they were deeper than the width of my hand. This condition is so easy to prevent that is not understandable how it can happen so often and so severely.

Treatment:

Prevention is the best treatment. When a collar is purchased for a dog, the collar needs to be checked frequently to see how tight or loose it is. If the collar is on a growing dog, the dog will grow, but the collar will not. The collar needs to be replaced and checked frequently. Do not put rubber bands, ropes, chains, wires, or cords on any animal; they will cause severe and unnecessary trauma. Just do not do it. If a collar or other device becomes embedded, you need to take your dog to the veterinarian.

Immunizations

Your pet should get all of its required immunizations from your veterinarian. It does not make any sense to have your pet get a disease that could have been prevented by immunization. You can find immunizations, such as those given by Luv My Pet, at low cost. It is so important that you have this done. Your veterinarian will know what vaccines are important for your area of the country. Rabies is, in most states, a required vaccination. Since cats are the pet most often not vaccinated for rabies, they are more likely to get rabies. Get it done if you have not done so—and keep them up-to-date.

Treatment:

You can obtain all vaccinations—besides rabies—from most feed stores and immunize them yourself.

Immunization Reactions

Immunization reactions are rather common and seem to occur mostly in the smaller breeds of dogs. The normal scenario is that the dog receives its vaccinations and, after thirty minutes or an hour, the dog becomes lethargic, has pale mucus membranes, vomits, or has a bowel movement, and lies still. All or a portion of these signs may be observed. Furthermore, some dogs will require hospitalization and have to be given intravenous fluids. This is not common but does occur on some occasions.

Treatment:

If your dog has a reaction at the immunization clinic, have it treated there. Normally Benadryl is injected or children's Benadryl is given orally. After 3–5 ccs of children's Benadryl, most dogs will recover within fifteen to twenty minutes, although some animals will take longer. You also have time on your side; as time passes, the immunization reaction dissipates. However, animals with severe reactions may require hospitalization. I have observed all of the above, so be aware. Normally nothing happens. If you give your own vaccines, you need to be aware, and you should have Benadryl handy for reactions that can and do occur. Of course, we hope that the Benadryl will not be needed.

Impacted Anal Glands or Scooting the Rear End on the Floor

It is not uncommon for an owner to find a dog scooting its bottom on the floor. There are two causes for this condition. One is caused by an excess of small segments of tapeworms (proglottids) around the anus that cause the need to scratch (pruritus). The other condition—and from my experience, the most frequent cause of this syndrome—is overfilled (impacted) anal glands.

Treatment:

The glands can be found and expressed very easily by placing a disposable-gloved index finger into the anus and feeling an enlargement or swelling at about the five o'clock and seven o'clock position. To feel both glands, you will have to shift your arm and hand or use the other hand to feel the other gland. They are expressed by squeezing the gland between the index finger that is in the anus and the thumb of the same hand. It is a darn good idea to have a Kleenex in your hand as you squeeze the gland since it will most often secrete a very pungent fluid. If the Kleenex is not in position, it will be all over you or your clothes and the smell is not good. These glands are the same anatomical glands that skunks use to spray.

Lameness

Most lameness is beyond your ability to change. However, you might be able to help a little with the pain. Small dog breeds tend to have luxating patellas, which can be moved back and forth out of joint. You will note the dog carrying its rear leg up and then walking normally, indicating that the patella is moving in and out of the proper position for the patella. Medium-sized dogs tend to have elbow dysplasia and large dog hip dysplasia—neither of which you can see—but you can observe an abnormal gait. When your pet walks, you may notice a lameness in one or more legs. If it is a small dog and you notice rear leg lameness, you can straighten its leg, grasp the patella, and move it in and out of joint. Do not be a gorilla during this procedure—be gentle. You cannot see the elbow dysplasia, but you might elicit pain in the area. Hip dysplasia—lameness of the hips—can become arthritic and more painful. Your treatment will be early and palliative and not curative for any of these conditions.

Treatment:

Aspirin can be given to help. It is best to give with food for a large dog. An adult aspirin can be given or dog aspirin can be purchased at pet stores. Smaller dogs do not need a full adult aspirin, but you can purchase smaller-dose aspirin at many stores. If all you have is adult aspirin, give the small dog half an aspirin. At first, it might take daily treatment, but then it will be every other day. The goal is to find a dose as low as possible and as infrequent as possible, but still aid the pet. We hope to see a reduction of the pain. Beyond this, you will need to see that special dog doctor.

Self-Trauma and Self-Mutilation

This is a condition that occurs when a dog or cat constantly chews or bites at parts of the body—most notably a foot, leg, or tail. Unfortunately, there is little you can do as an owner. There are several causes that can make this phenomenon occur. The one that you can perhaps help is the psychological aspect of this disease. Changes in daily routine, introduction of new surroundings, new carpets, moving to new surroundings, or a family member leaving are all possibilities for initiation of this condition. This is not an easy disease to overcome. I have seen this condition occur when a first child is born and the attention is directed away from the dog. The dog may self-mutilate or vomit to gain attention. Bandaging normally does not help since the dog or cat will have the bandage off before you get out the door.

Treatment:

Sometimes a change in the space the animal has to play or run will overcome the self-mutilation. A farm or acreage of land has been helpful—as is training or spending more time with the dog. This is a trial-and-error proposition if you have the patience and time to do so.

Seizures

Since there are many causes of seizures, these syndromes are best left for your pet's doctor to properly diagnose. The most common seizures are those that originate in the brain, but, fortunately, there are some things you can do. If your pet has a seizure, you need to know that there is nothing you can do to stop it. You may notice your pet acting odd just before the seizure and then the animal will start convulsing. Normally, seizures last for short periods. If a seizure is prolonged, it is an emergency and you need to take your pet to the veterinarian as soon as possible. It is not uncommon for a dog to have seizures two or three times in one month. The unfortunate thing about this type of seizure is that, even on medicine, your pet can seize. It may have two or three seizure per month while receiving treatments. The doctor may or may not dispense medicine since he or she knows that the medicine will do only so much. However, if the pet is convulsing more frequently, medicine will normally be dispensed. Do not expect it to completely eliminate seizure activity—it is a lifetime palliative treatment.

Treatment:

There is no over-the-counter treatment that can be recommended. The information is provided here for those who have or may experience seizures in pets.

Toenails Trimmed and Bleeding

If you have ever trimmed toenails, you have probably had the joy of bleeding toenails. It can be quite frustrating, but you can prevent it by studying the toenail and noting that the end of the toenail has a smaller diameter. As you get closer to the toe, the nail becomes larger in diameter. If you make your cut on the smaller diameter of the toenail, you normally will not cause bleeding. I must emphasize *normally* because you might occasionally get some bleeding, assuming that you did not happen to cut on the larger diameter of the toenail. If you do cause bleeding by cutting too high, you can use the following treatment to stop the bleeding.

Treatment:

Purchase some cornstarch and keep it handy as you cut toenails. If you cause toenail bleeding, hold the cornstarch next to the bleeding toenail, apply a small amount of pressure, and you will have stopped the bleeding.

What Food Should I Feed?

I am often asked what to feed pets. In this modern age, dog and cat foods are all pretty good, and you can find folks and feed salesmen who will say food such-and-such is best. We personally like and feed Hill's Science Diet to our cat, and the cat does very well. The test of any diet is how well the animal is doing. Is the weight okay? Is the hair coat okay? Are there any issues with digestion? Does the dog or cat like what is being fed? If so, then you are on the right track. This is not rocket science. If you fulfill the above things, you're doing the right things. The big issue is not to overfeed and be aware of your pet's weight and overall health. Remember that it is your job to monitor your pet's health.

Treatment:

Almost any pet food that you purchase at a pet store, tractor store, grocery store, or feed store will meet your requirements. Most often, the better pet foods will list meat as the first ingredient. Vegetable diets are not recommended for dogs and cats because they do not provide the proper nutrition.

Chapter 2:
Behavioral Problems

From now on, ending a sentence with a preposition is something up with which I will not put.
—*Sir Winston Churchill*

Some of the most frustrating issues with our pets are those over which we seem to have the least control. They appear hard to overcome, but, as with many things, when we have knowledge, frustration seems to melt like snow.

Messing in the House or Defecating on Floors

This is a frustrating condition and requires lots of patience and training to overcome. You may need to seek professional help to get completely rid of this condition, but most likely with patience, consistency, and persistence, you will prevail.

Treatment:

Patience, patience, patience is necessary. Do not punish the animal for dirtying the floor. Take the pet outside frequently and normally on a leash so that you can be close to the animal when the animal goes to the bathroom. Reward the dog with a small treat and praise the pet with lots of attaboys. Take the dog outside frequently—as often as you possibly can—to help prevent accidents. The treats need not be large; small training treats are available at pet stores. Cats are not as prone to this type of training. I know of some cats that were in the house 100 percent of the time. They soiled the floor even though the litter box was cleaned frequently. It is imperative that the litter be cleared very frequently. This is why I like the automatic-cleaning litter boxes. They work well with one or two cats, but will not work with numerous cats. Sometimes letting the cat become an indoor-outdoor cat can resolve the issue. However, you have to be willing to let the cat out. Note: Lots of cats get lost and end up as strays, so be aware.

Petting-Induced Aggression in Cats

Petting-induced aggression occurs while you are petting a cat and the cat suddenly attacks and bites—sometimes quite hard. As you become acquainted with this syndrome, you will notice when the cat is about to bite you. It might bolt off the couch or just sit and look at you as your hand or arm is bleeding. I am not sure of the etiology of this or why only some cats do it, but it is an annoying phenomena. It is prudent to advise guests not to pet your cat so that they don't get bitten. Some guests will think that you're kidding until they get bitten.

Treatment:

I have no OTC treatment for this condition other than to make you aware that this happens and that you should pet your cat for just a short time and then stop before you get bitten. Sometimes it will bite when you stop petting, so get up, move, sit back down, and leave the cat alone.

Urine Spraying in Cats

This marking of territory occurs when the cat stands with tail upright, spraying urine horizontally onto objects or walls. Often the cat will not use the litter box. Spraying can become a form of inappropriate behavior. It turns out that urine spraying is the most common behavioral problem in cats. Male and female cats will both spray; the most common time a female will spray is during her heat period (estrus). A higher incidence of feline spraying is during indoor confinement. Neutering of male cats has proven to be quite effective. A majority of neutered male cats stops spraying immediately, but others take a few months. Spaying female cats is not as effective as neutering males, but it helps reduce spraying. If your cat has been confined to the house, sometimes letting the cat out may stop inappropriate defecation and urination. When you clean a violated area, use an ammonia product as the final wipe cleaner—often this will stop the soiling in that area. It is not 100 percent guaranteed, but it is sure worth a try.

Treatment:

Clean the litter box frequently. The automatic-cleaning boxes help with this. If you are not home, it cleans shortly after the cat leaves the litter box. The more frequently one can change the litter, the better. Of course, neutering is not an OTC treatment, but it seems to be quite effective and you should give this treatment serious consideration.

Skunk-Sprayed Dog or Cat

Dogs and cats seem to be very inquisitive when it comes to some wildlife—and skunks are no exception. Since skunks have few predators, they tend to get into our neighborhoods and do their thing. They can spray pets—and get them well. The pets come home smelling like a skunk. The treatment is quite simple and you can purchase the ingredients at any grocery store. After mixing the items or compounds, use it all up. Do not attempt to store the leftovers since it is a very unstable mixture. You can sponge or pour the treatment onto the dog or cat.

Treatment:

To mix up your skunk treatments, follow these simple steps:

1. The mixture will need to be in a clean bucket or a large bowl. Do not mix in a bottle or small container because the ingredients are very active.
2. Add one quart of hydrogen peroxide to one quart of water.
3. Add ¼ cup of Arm & Hammer baking soda (sodium bicarbonate).
4. Add 1–2 teaspoons of liquid soap (dish or laundry soap is okay).
5. Mix with a plastic utensil.
6. Protect your eyes—and the pet's eyes. An ointment can be obtained at the pharmacy to put into the pet's eyes before pouring the solution.
7. Use rubber gloves to protect your hands.
8. Clean the dog after ten minutes and double-check its eyes to make sure they are okay. You may not get 100 percent off the face, but you will get the majority if you are careful with your sponge.
9. Discard any excess solution.

Feces-Eating (Coprophagy)

Coprophagia or feces-eating is the ingestion of feces by the dog or cat. It is common in dogs, but is rather rare in cats. There have been many theories about why this occurs, but the bottom line is that no one really knows why or what triggers this type of behavior. This condition should not be considered abnormal. There are normally few deleterious consequences associated with dogs or cats eating feces other than severe bad breath. Sometimes dogs will ingest the feces of other animals.

Treatment:

Picking up feces as it is produced is the most effective treatment. When the product is not available to eat, it cannot be consumed. Some animals will respond to foods that have so-called proteolytic enzymes such as pineapple, figs, and squash. Sprinkling a bit of meat tenderizer on the dog's food may help. Anti-coprophagia tablets are available at Pet Smart and Petco. Different things work differently in different animals. Although I have not found the pills to be very effective, you might be lucky and have great success.

Chapter 3:
Intestinal Disorders

We set sail on the new sea because there is knowledge to be gained.
—John F. Kennedy

So many of the conditions found in dogs and cats that involve intestinal disorders are frequently the same signs noted in people. These syndromes are easily recognized due to obvious signs and similar symptoms in man. The issue is not the problem, but how to handle the problem. Here some simple solutions available for resolution of many of these issues.

Bad Breath (Halitosis)

Bad breath can be caused by a lot of different things, including coprophagia. Offering soft foods will add to a pet's bad breath. Soft foods can also cause the teeth to become caked with food. Both soft and hard pet foods can and do cause teeth to rot when they are allowed to accumulate on the teeth. A few years ago, teeth in pets were almost completely ignored, but now it is recognized that such things add to the disease-process in animals in many ways. Since there is no panacea for this condition, the following will give you some help in reducing bad breath, but is not a cure.

Treatment:

Hard, dry foods will help to break away the food accumulated on the teeth. This will not completely solve the problem, but it will help. The other issue is to brush the teeth with a toothbrush. A new product called ProDen Plaque Off® for animals has been shown to be effective against bad breath, tartar, and plaque. The product can be purchased at www.international-dental.com, (909) 646-9949, or info@international-dental.com. The cost is low and, if directions are followed, a small container will last about a year. Another product, Tartar Shield, can be purchased from your veterinarian or online at www.tartarshield.com . I have found the product to be well received by pets and it does a good job. Give it a try—I think you will like it if your pet has bad breath.

Constipation

Constipation, an impaction of the intestines, can be due to lack of mobility of the gut, diet, dehydration, and numerous other causes that require attention from your veterinarian. We will focus on improper diet and dehydration. Concentrated bone diets are sure to cause constipation, which is not easy to clear. Dry food with limited access to water is another cause. There are many other issues in dogs and cats, but none are treatable with over-the-counter drugs.

Treatment:

Give a warm water mineral oil enema and change to a more nutritious diet. If necessary, Vaseline or mineral oil can be given orally or an enema will do the trick. In cats, feeding Carnation canned milk has also been very effective.

Passing Intestinal Gas (Flatulence)

There are many causes of intestinal gas, but we will only cover those simple things that you can do something about. Intestinal gas comes from four major causes: swallowing air (aerophagia), bacterial fermentation, gas diffusion from the blood to the intestines, and acids and bases in the digestive tract. Diets high in fiber and soybean meal can be the major cause of flatulence in your pet. Cat diets containing large amounts of lactose may be the culprit.

If this is a great problem in your pet, a trial of hypoallergenic food for three to four weeks might resolve or help improve the gas production and prove or disprove a digestive allergy. Many other causes of flatulence are best left to your favorite pet doctor.

Treatment:

Aerophagia can be difficult to overcome, but it may be aided by feeding more frequent, smaller amounts of food. Since dogs tend to gulp their food down, this reduces the amount of air taken into the stomach that must pass through the intestines. Low-fiber diets may help resolve the issue, but there is no pixie dust that will make it go away. You have to give it a try and see how it goes—the best of luck to you. There are several OTC items that are designed to treat flatulence and some may be of benefit. If you have a real issue, you might try some of them such as Gas-X.

Hairballs

Since cats tend to lick their bodies, they ingest hair. The hair that is ingested creates some problems in some cats. Treat the cat every so often to prevent any really bad issue from occurring due to excess hair in the digestive system.

Treatment:

Pet stores have tubes of compounds that can be smeared on the cat's nose and feet to be licked off to treat the hairballs. Also, Carnation's canned milk can be fed to the cat. The concentration of both of these compounds will draw water into the intestinal tract and cause the cat to have a loose or soft stool that will move the hair out of the intestinal tract.

Loose Stools

Loose stools have many causes, but you will not know the cause of the loose stools. Diarrhea is when the animal has stool after stool that is loose. When dehydration occurs due to the loss of fluids, fluids must be replaced. To determine whether the dog or cat has dehydration associated with the loose stools, grab some loose skin, pull it up, and let go. If it pops right back down, the pet probably does not have dehydration. If the skin is somewhat slow going back down, the pet probably has about 4–6 percent dehydration. If the skin is quite slow going back down, it could be 6–8 percent dehydration. If the skin stays up and the eyes are sunken back in the head, it may be 10–12 percent or more. At this point, your pet is at risk of death and should see a veterinarian as soon as possible. Actually, the pet should have seen its doctor before it got to this condition.

Among the most common causes of loose stools are hookworms and coccidia (a cellular parasite), and in younger pets, possibly parvovirus. If your pet has loose stools, before starting any treatment, look at its gums. Are they pale or white? If so, the loose stools or diarrhea may be due to these parasites. If the gums are pale or white, go directly to your veterinarian because your pet may need a blood transfusion. If you are unsure of the cause, I recommend that you treat for both internal parasites and loose stools. *At a minimum, you should have stool samples run to determine whether or not your pet has intestinal parasites.*

Treatment:

Imodium can be purchased OTC at a Walmart, grocery store, pharmacy, or other store. **Note:** *Collies and related breeds may be overly sensitive to loperamide.*

- Imodium (loperamide): The tablets or caplets are two milligram tablets and liquid 1 mg in 7.5 cc.

Dosage: The following dose regimen will normally overcome loose stools:

- Small dog (under ten pounds): One tablet twice daily for three days, but no longer than five days.
- Medium size (ten to thirty pounds): Two tablets twice daily for three days, but no longer than five days.
- Large dog (over thirty pounds): Three tablets twice daily for three days, but no longer than five days.

Do not overdose! Dogs will act drugged if you give too much. Be very careful going beyond three days of treatment in a dog or a cat. Watch for cessation of the loose stools. Even if infected with parasites, the loperamide will slow down the loose stools and treatment for parasites at the same time, often eliminating the cause of the loose stools, hastening healing.

Puppies:

If they have loose stools, they probably have hookworms or other parasites. You can slow down the loose stools with liquid Imodium (loperamide). However, if you value the puppy's health, it should be taken to your veterinarian. Liquid Imodium normally has 1 mg in 7.5 cc or 2 mg in 15 cc.

Puppy Dosage:

Give 1.25 ml (1/4 teaspoon) of liquid Imodium (a teaspoon is 5 ml, half a teaspoon is 2.5 ml, and ¼ teaspoon is 1.25 ml).

Cats:

Debate rages about the use of loperamide in cats. However, it has been used successfully. Many doctors will not recommend use of this drug in cats. I have used it many times without issue. However, this does not prevent an unexpected reaction from occurring if this drug is used in cats. Also treating for internal parasites is indicated along with the loperamide. Any drug used in any species can—and has or might—cause adverse responses or reactions.

Cat Dose:

- Adult cats: One 2 mg tablet or capsule once daily for three days.
- Cats less than five pounds: 1 mg or half of a 2 mg tablet once daily for three days.
- Kittens: Use liquid Imodium and give 1/8 teaspoon once daily for three days.

Watch for response. If stools form, reduce or stop the loperamide, but continue the parasite treatments.

Pepto-Bismol: Can be purchased at grocery stores, Walmart, or pharmacies. Pepto-Bismol can be used at the same time that loperamide (Imodium) is being given. Black stools can be caused by Pepto-Bismol or by upper-intestinal bleeding. Be aware when you use Pepto-Bismol that it is the drug, not blood.

- Small Dogs (under ten pounds): One tablet twice daily for three days.
- Medium Dogs (ten to thirty pounds): Two tablets twice daily for three days.
- Large Dogs (Thirty pounds and up): Three tablets twice daily for three days.

Note: Do not use Pepto-Bismol in cats because it contains aspirin-like compounds (salicylates). Cats do not tolerate this compound well and you could accidentally kill your cat.

Persistent Loose Stools:

Many dog and cats examined by me have had every possible drug for loose stools. The following diet has worked very well in incurable loose stools (diarrhea). Give it a try, but you must follow the directions completely to be effective. If your pet has intestinal cancer, most treatments are not effective. This diet has been given for several weeks without any known issues. *It is important that no other foods be fed while using the following diet* to control loose stools. This diet should be followed for at least three weeks.

This is a very effective treatment—but follow directions closely. No other food of any type can be fed, including all treats, etc.

Cottage cheese and rice diet for diarrhea

- The formula is one cup of instant rice to four ounces of cottage cheese.
- Since most people will not fix only one cup of rice, the minimum normally is four cups of rice.
- Fix four cups of instant rice and let it cool in the refrigerator.
- After the rice is cool, mix sixteen ounces of cottage cheese with the rice.
- Feed the rice and cottage cheese to the pet.
- The rice and cottage cheese that is not being fed should be kept in the refrigerator.

Meat-Exclusive Diets

All exclusive meat diets (muscle meats) are detrimental to your pet's health. The mechanism for these phenomena has to do with the blood calcium and phosphorus levels. When a critter is fed an all-meat diet, the bones will eventually be absorbed, causing the bones to become very thin. When the bones become very thin, there is a high probability that the bones in your pet will start to break—either by what seem to be unexplained causes or from very slight trauma.

If you have fed some vegetables along with the all-meat diet, I have found that this has or will result in prolonging the absorption of calcium from the bones. Some vegetables will not prevent the thinning of bones when the major food provided is striated muscle meats. Normally, owners are shocked when they learn that their pet has this syndrome. Owners normally think that they are being kind to the animal, but they are actually killing it.

In addition to the bone issues, animals often develop diarrhea and dandruff before the bones break. This phenomenon has been well documented by Mark M. Morris Jr. of Hill's Science Diet fame. In the February 15, 1971, issue of the *American Veterinary Medical Association Journal,* he described the events that occur as a result of all-meat diets. In "The Effects of the Exclusive Feeding of an All-Meat Dog Food," he showed that an all-meat diet can kill a dog in three months. I have seen bones as thin as a sheet of paper in dogs fed chicken, turkey, and beef all-meat diets.

Do not—under any circumstances—follow an all-meat diet. If you do, you are guaranteed a trip to the veterinarian—maybe even to put your pet to sleep. It is just a matter of time. If the bones break, they may be so thin that any attempt to fix them will make the situation worse. This syndrome of all striated muscle meats may be the cause of the death of your pet.

Treatment:

Do not feed all-meat diets. If you have been following an all-meat diet, stop and purchase normal pet food.

Motion Sickness
Or Traveling with Pets

I have been asked many times to give pets a sedative for traveling. First, if you have traveled with your pet and the pet does well, you do not need anything for the pet on your trip. Because treatment is so readily available in grocery stores and pharmacies, there is no need to start with treatment. Get started on the trip and take the medicine along with you or just stop in the next town and pick it up. If you're going on a long flight to Hawaii or a foreign country, there is no sedative on the planet that will treat the animal for the duration of the trip—so don't do it. I was assigned to one duty station when dogs were sedated. While they were on the tarmac waiting to be loaded onto the aircraft, the dogs died due to the heat and central nervous system depression due to drugs.

Treatment:

Benadryl is the OTC treatment of choice. The dosage depends on the size of the pet. Give 1–2 mg per pound of body weight. Besides the liquid, the compound comes in 2, 4, and 25 mg tablets. Perhaps the tablets are easier to administer so you can choose whichever you prefer. I would start with 1 mg per pound and see how that works since it is easy to add but hard to subtract once the medication is given.

Remember: Start your travel without medication and if necessary give the medicine. The dosage charts are low-dose, so start with the low dose since every animal responds differently. If you feel the animal needs more, repeat the dose.

Benadryl 1 and 2 mg
First-Dose Chart Available Over-the-Counter in Grocery Stores
Repeat Dose if Necessary

	Dose 1 mg tablets	Weight Pounds	Dose 2 mg tablets
1	¼ or .25	1	See 1 mg dose
2	½ or .5	2	See 1 mg dose
3	1	3	See 1 mg dose
4	1.5	4	See 1 mg dose
5	1.75	5	See 1 mg dose
6	2	6	1
7	3	7	1.5
8	3	8	1.5
9	4	9	2
10	4	10	2
11	5	11	2.5
12	Do not use	12	3
13	Do not use	13	3
14	Do not use	14	3.5
15	Do not use	15	3.5
16	Do not use	16	4

17	Do not use	17	4
18	Do not use	18	4
19	Do not use	19	5
20	Do not use	20	5

Benadryl 25 Mg First Dose Chart
Available Over-The-Counter in Drug Stores
Repeat Dose If Necessary

Weight Pounds	Dose * # of tablets	Weight Pounds	Dose # of tablets	Weight Pounds	Dose # of tablets	Weight Pounds	Dose # of tablets
21	.5	41	1	61	2	81	2
22	.5	42	1	62	2	82	2
23	.5	43	1	63	2	83	2
24	.5	44	1	64	2	84	2
25	1	45	1	65	2	85	2
26	1	46	1	66	2	86	2
27	1	47	1	67	2	87	2
28	1	48	1	68	2	88	2
29	1	49	1	69	2	89	2
30	1	50	1	70	2	90	2.5
31	1	51	1.5	71	2	91	2.5
32	1.25	52	1.5	72	2	92	2.5
33	1.25	53	1.5	73	2	93	2.5
34	1.25	54	1.5	74	2	94	2.5
35	1.25	55	1.5	75	2	95	2.5
36	1.25	56	1.5	76	2	96	2.5
37	1.25	57	1.5	77	2	97	3
38	1.25	58	1.5	78	2	98	3
39	1.25	59	2	79	2	99	3
40	1.25	60	2	80	2	100	3

*1=1 tablet, .25 = ¼ tablet, .5 = ½ tablet, .75 = ½ + ¼ tablets.

Intestinal Parasites

Hookworms, roundworms, whipworms, tapeworms, and coccidian are the most common—but by no means all—of the internal parasites. We will discuss the most common ones.

Intestinal parasites include hookworms and roundworms, which have a migration phase in the body. Whipworms develop in the lower intestine. Coccidia develop in the cells of the intestine and break out, causing diarrhea and intestinal bleeding. Hookworms can also cause bloody, black stools. Due to loss of blood caused by hookworms and coccidian, the gums of your pet may become pale to white. Your pet may also become dehydrated and lethargic or stop eating. The paler the gums become, the worse the infection of the hookworms or coccidian. The whiter the gums become, the more of an emergency, which necessitates good treatment and perhaps a quick need to see your veterinarian. Pale or white gums could also mean that your pet is suffering from dehydration. They are easily treated with compounds available at pet and feed stores. I recommend a combination of Pyrantel and Praziquantel. It is readily available and the treatment dosage recommendations for the compounds are included with the package. Be sure not to overdose.

Tapeworms normally come from fleas on the animal's body. When the dog or cat bites at the flea, it is swallowed and the tapeworm develops from the flea. The flea is called an intermediate host and the flea has the tapeworm egg in its body. You will see wiggling, rice-looking things on the feces or around the anus of the animal. If so, use either the Pyrantel-Praziquantel combination or Praziquantel to treat your dog or cat. These drug names can be found on the label of the product. It is easy to ask the people at the store for the product by name. They will be able to locate it and price it for you. It comes in multiple doses per container. I have found that some feed stores will sell one dose—ask if you do not want to purchase the entire package.

If you are treating your pet for hookworms or roundworms, you should repeat the treatment in two or three weeks to get the parasites that were in migration—and not in the intestinal tract—the first time you treated. After the second treatment, it is a good idea to have a fecal sample tested to make sure that you got all the worms. If there are still signs of parasites, treat again.

- **Ivermectin:** This product—purchased at tractor stores or feed stores—can also be used for hookworms and roundworms. The dosage recommendations can be found in the chart under the discussion on external parasites. Ivermectin is safe for pregnant pets; however, it has been recommended not to be used in puppies less than six weeks of age. Despite this, I have treated many small puppies for scabies with this product without any harm to the puppy. This product can be given orally or injected under the skin. Either way is just as effective. Ivermectin is extremely safe to use. One would have to administer ten to fifteen times the dosage indicated in the table, "1 Percent" Ivermectin Dosing Chart" on page 45 in order to bring harm to an animal. *Since Collie-bred dogs with a special gene defect allow more Ivermectin into the central nervous system than other breeds, it is not considered a good idea to give Ivermectin to these breeds or any that are related to these breeds.*

- **Coccidia:** Your veterinarian can best treat this condition, but if you fail to see your veterinarian, you can follow these instructions. The doses to use are 25 mg per pound on day one and 12.5 mg per pound for days two through five. Feed stores have a solution called Sulmet® which is Sulfadimethoxine. It is a 12.5 percent solution, which is the same as 125 mg per cc. Perhaps you have or are using this solution and did not know the proper dosage to use. *If you overdose with sulfur drugs, you can cause dry eye in your pet. I believe it best to let your veterinarian do this for you.* If you refuse to see your veterinarian, you can use the following dosage schedule.

Treatment Charts for Day 1 and Days 2–5

The dosage recommendation in the charts is based on the 125 mg or 12.5 percent solution of Sulmet® (Sulfadimethoxine). Sulfadimethoxine is the compound used to treat coccidia in dogs and cats. However, the solution Sulmet® is designed to be put into the water of chickens for treatment of coccidia, which is the same drug used in dogs and cats to treat coccidia. The Sulmet® comes in a rather large container; if you use it, you probably will have no further use for it. The charts have the dose using Sulmet® liquid in ccs. Without the use of a microscope to examine a fecal flotation, it will be very difficult for you to know what you are treating. It is for this reason we encourage you to take your pet to your veterinarian for diagnosis and treatment of this disease. At the minimum, you should have a fecal run to see if there is even a need for this treatment. As stated earlier, we know that many of you will not—and have not—taken your pet to see a veterinarian, and we realize that you may not in this case or even in the future. *Do not overdose with this compound. If you do, you are almost assured that you will have eye issues as a result of the overdose.*

Day 1 Dose

12.5 Percent Sulmet (Sulfadimethoxine 125 Mg) Dosing Day 1 Chart
(Weight Divided by 5 = Dose in CCs)
Give by Mouth Only

Dilute with Water and Double the Volume

Weight Pounds	Dose CCS	Weight Pounds	Dose CCS	Weight Pounds	Dose CCS	Weight Pounds	Dose CCS
1	0.2	21	4.2	41	8.2	61	12.2
2	0.4	22	4.4	42	8.4	62	12.4
3	0.6	23	4.6	43	8.6	63	12.6
4	0.8	24	4.8	44	8.8	64	12.8
5	1.0	25	5.0	45	9.0	65	13.0
6	1.2	26	5.2	46	9.2	66	13.2
7	1.4	27	5.4	47	9.4	67	13.4
8	1.6	28	5.6	48	9.6	68	13.6
9	1.8	29	5.8	49	9.8	69	13.8
10	2.0	30	6.0	50	10.0	70	14.0
11	2.2	31	6.2	51	10.2	71	14.2
12	2.4	32	6.4	52	10.4	72	14.4
13	2.6	33	6.6	53	10.6	73	14.6
14	2.8	34	6.8	54	10.8	74	14.8
15	3.0	35	7.0	55	11.0	75	15.0
16	3.2	36	7.2	56	11.2	76	15.2
17	3.4	37	7.4	57	11.4	77	15.4
18	3.6	38	7.6	58	11.6	78	15.6
19	3.8	39	7.8	59	11.8	79	15.8
20	4.0	40	8.0	60	12.0	80	16.0

Weight Pounds	Dose CCS
81	16.2
82	16.4
83	16.6
84	16.8
85	17.0
86	17.2
87	17.4
88	17.6
89	17.8
90	18.0
91	18.2
92	18.4
93	18.6
94	18.8
95	19.0
96	19.2
97	19.4
98	19.6
99	19.8
100	20.0

Day 2–5 Dose

12.5 Percent Sulmet (Sulfadimethoxine 125 Mg) Dosing Day 2–5 Chart
(Divide Day 1 Dose by 2 = Dose in CCs)
Give by Mouth Only

Dilute With Water and Double the Volume

Weight Pounds	Dose ccs	Weight Pounds	Dose ccs	Weight Pounds	Dose ccs	Weight Pounds	Dose ccs	Weight Pounds	Dose ccs
1	0.1	21	2.1	41	4.1	61	6.1	81	8.1
2	0.2	22	2.2	42	4.2	62	6.2	82	8.2
3	0.3	23	2.3	43	4.3	63	6.3	83	8.3
4	0.4	24	2.4	44	4.4	64	6.4	84	8.4
5	0.5	25	2.5	45	4.5	65	6.5	85	8.5
6	0.6	26	2.6	46	4.6	66	6.6	86	8.6
7	0.7	27	2.7	47	4.7	67	6.7	87	8.7
8	0.8	28	2.8	48	4.8	68	6.8	88	8.8
9	0.9	29	5.8	49	4.9	69	6.9	89	8.9
10	1.0	30	3.0	50	5.0	70	7.0	90	9.0
11	1.1	31	3.1	51	5.1	71	7.1	91	9.1
12	1.2	32	3.2	52	5.2	72	7.2	92	9.2
13	1.3	33	3.3	53	5.3	73	7.3	93	9.3
14	1.4	34	3.4	54	5.4	74	7.4	94	9.4
15	1.5	35	3.5	55	5.5	75	7.5	95	9.5
16	1.6	36	3.6	56	5.6	76	7.6	96	9.6
17	1.7	37	3.7	57	5.7	77	7.7	97	9.7
18	1.8	38	3.8	58	5.8	78	7.8	98	9.8
19	1.9	39	3.9	59	5.9	79	7.9	99	9.9
20	2.0	40	4.0	60	6.0	80	8.0	100	10.0

Vomiting

As with diarrhea, vomiting can be a serious issue that can rapidly cause dehydration in your pet. There are many causes of vomiting, including foreign bodies, cloth, plastic, coins, knives, and cancer. There are many other causes that we will leave for you to take to your veterinarian. Some are rather innocent; it is the innocent vomiting that we will cover in this book.

Cats will often pig out, but a few minutes after eating, will throw up the food as though it was pushed out of a tube on to the floor—or more likely on your favorite rug. This is not a disease issue; it is the owner putting too much food into the bowl.

Dogs and cats that have eaten grass or other plants will also be stimulated to vomit, but there is no disease present. The reason for grass and other plant consumption by dogs and cats remains a mystery. Many theories have been proposed and I have been asked and told many reasons for this phenomenon. Your suggestion may be as good as anyone else's, but the real reason is unknown.

Another cause can be certain medicines that are given orally. Within a few minutes, the cat or dog will vomit the medicine and either clear or yellow fluids. The clear fluid is from the stomach and the yellow fluid is from the duodenum.

Treatment:

If your cat is throwing up food after eating, you should reduce the amount of food it is being feed. If you are giving medicines and the animal is having issue keeping it down, then thirty to forty minutes before giving the medicine, give the pet Pepcid AC: the cat gets a quarter-tablet, small dogs a half-tablet, and large dog a full tablet. Famotidine by any brand or generic name will work as well.

Chapter 4:
Skin Conditions

I like pigs. Dogs look up to us. Cats look down on us. Pigs treat us as equals.
—*Sir Winston Churchill*

Skin conditions range from the intriguing to the obscure to the obvious. Let's look at perhaps the most obvious. Skin is a living tissue that protects, heals, stretches, dries, moistens, and aids in the appearances of our pets, but it can be a challenge to overcome some minor and terrible conditions. We see here a few of these conditions that can be properly treated with over-the-counter medicines.

Allergic Response to Plastic Feeding Bowls

A rather common finding in dogs is caused by owners purchasing plastic feeding bowls. The lips and area around the dog's mouth turn red due to inflammation that is quite sore. At times, it can get so bad that fluids are being expelled from the affected area. I have seen some cases that were ignored so long that the lips and area around the mouth were almost fire-engine red in response to the plastic bowls used for feeding.

Treatment:

Do not use plastic feeding bowls. If you are, dispose of the plastic bowls so that you do not cause this problem in your dog. If your dog has this syndrome, wash with a mild soap and water and apply hydrocortisone cream. It is best treated by your favorite veterinarian since he or she can add other medicines that will aid in healing the lesion quickly.

Barbering:
Excessive Grooming of Cats

Cats will sometimes lick all the hair off of part of their body. I have no idea what stimulates this condition. However, when you see this, it will be an area that is easy for the cat to lick. A cat tongue is such that it takes the hair off like a barber's clippers. The skin in the area always seems to be normal and the edges of the area are normally straight. It is normally square or rectangular. The treatment for this condition is to keep the cat somewhat sedated. I do not agree with that approach. Who wants a pet moping around half asleep or doped up? My wife and I have had a cat that would do this. In time, she would leave it alone and the hair would grow back in. The cat did not look good with the hair missing from its abdomen and we did not want others to see her in that condition. But it is what it is and it does recover. Everything else about the cat was absolutely normal. Early on, it was thought to be an endocrine syndrome, but it was only excessive grooming. Be patient and it eventually grows back.

Treatment:

Leave it alone it will come back when the cat stops licking the area.

Biting Flies

Flies do not bite. Their proboscis has a rough end that they use to scrape against the skin, causing raw areas on the margins of the ear.

It frequently occurs on the ears because the area has limited hair. This condition can be very painful to the pet. The main thing is to remove the dog from its environment and, if possible, put the dog in a dark area since flies do not normally enter dark areas. If the dog is not removed from the environment, it will become worse or reoccur. Since these flies work on the eyes of cattle, farm dogs *may* be more prone to exposure than other pets.

Treatment:

Clean the ears frequently and apply topical ointment. Triple antibiotic ointments are available in grocery stores and pharmacies. One treatment will not work—the ears must be cleaned and treated daily.

Demodex
Red Mange Hair Loss

We see tons of this disease in our facility. Since many people ignore their pet's health, the cases we see are so far advanced with secondary bacterial infection that it is unbelievable. It is disgusting that people would allow such conditions, but unfortunately they do. The mite is in the follicle of the hairs. When viewed under microscope, they appear somewhat cigar-shaped with little legs and feet. They are disgusting little critters. The red skin in this condition is due to the mites, and, unfortunately, shows at an advanced stage of the disease. In addition, the dog will have a distinct smell that—once identified—can be diagnosed from the look and smell. It can be treated today, but a few years ago, we had to put such animals to sleep since there was no treatment.

Treatment:

For this condition, we use Ivermectin. It can be injected under the skin or given by mouth, but is usually given orally. We have to calculate the dosage for every dog, but it is quite simple. Sometimes the treatment must be repeated, but normally it is treated within fifteen days. Retreatment will have to be determined by you since you are the one who sees the animal. If retreatment is necessary, continue the dosage for days 3–14. There have been cases that have needed three months of treatment. Be aware that it may not be a short treatment period.

How to Calculate Dosage:

WARNING: do not use these calculations unless your pet weighs twenty-five pounds. I have provided in this example how to calculate the proper dose for your pet based on its weight; please double-check your math before administering the drug. Let's use a twenty-five-pound dog in this example:

- For day one, divide the weight of the dog in pounds by 100. 25 pounds/100 =.25 CC. On Day 1, the dose is .25 cc (only ¼ of a cc or ml).
- On Day 2, double the Day 1 dose. The Day 2 dose would be .50 cc (½ cc or ml only).
- On Days 3–14, double the Day 2 dose so that the dose (1 cc) is given daily for the next twelve days.

Dull Hair Coat

The most probable cause or your pet's dull hair coat, excluding filth and dirt, is nutritional. You might consider changing diets. Most diets in this new millennium are quite good and most will provide your pet with a proper nutrition. However, if you feel that you want to make the hair coat on your pet look better, give this a try. While Dr. Mark M. Morris Jr. was studying the quality of consumer pet diets in 1971, he discovered that most diets had deficiencies and required some form of extra supplement. Since that time, pet foods are greatly improved, and these supplements are still valuable even today.

Treatment:

Add a tablespoon of Mazola® corn oil and a hardboiled egg to the dry food dog. Many folks tell me that they cannot afford an egg per day, so add one as often as you can.

Caution: Corn oil can cause and has caused loose stools in some dogs. If this happens, cut back to perhaps half a tablespoon, a quarter of a tablespoon, or whatever level your dog will tolerate. The egg for your pet's health must be hardboiled—*never* use a raw egg because they have avidin. This glycoprotein in the egg white ties up biotin, resulting in a Vitamin B deficiency in your dog. Be a part of the solution—not the problem. I have never tried fried or scrambled eggs—but be my guest to try it and write to me with your findings.

Fleas

I have chosen to treat fleas separately from the major topic of external parasites. I have had more people lie to me about their treatment of fleas on their pets—and had more people get mad at me when I tell them that their pet has fleas. I have decided to cover this subject all by itself. Fleas bite and eat blood and poop blood and leave little red bites on the belly of the dog. The classic signs of flea infestation need not be present to enable one to make a diagnosis. It is a huge misconception to think that the cat that never goes outside does not have fleas. People could not be more wrong on this issue.

Certain parts of the North America have no issue with fleas because of their higher elevations. It is actually a function of the ambient temperature, but at the higher elevation, there are no fleas. Fleas die when the temperature dips below 20 degrees Fahrenheit for more than forty-eight hours. In higher altitudes, you are more likely to see times when the temperatures fall. Fleas are not compatible with the weather conditions at high elevations. Fleas can transmit disease and cause anemia in your pet. Think about it—if your pet gets on your bed and you sleep there and you do not treat for fleas—you will have fleas in your bed. Wow! Exciting—don't you think?

The toxic sprays and dips that we used in the seventies and eighties are a thing of the past. It's pretty amazing to see the advancement the new topical treatments that require a once-a-month treatment between the animal's shoulder blades. It is just that simple. I have asked folks what they use to treat fleas and they tell me, but the poor critter is covered in fleas. I have developed a bias against some products. My favorite—and the one we use—is the prescription-required Revolution®. I will not recommend it because it is not an over-the-counter medicine and it requires a prescription. The recommended products are available from your veterinarian, feed stores, tractor stores, Petco, and Pet Smart.

Treatment:

I recommend the use of Advantage® for cat and Advantix® for dogs. Put the drug between the shoulder blades. We have used these products on thousands of animals and both products do a great job. There have been folks that happened to put dog Advantix on cats and there was no issue. However, if a cat licks the product, there can be considerable signs and lots of salivation. Some folks have told me that the product does not work. When questioned further, they have used it once every six months or every three months—it has to be used monthly. However, it is possible that the flea population you are treating may become resistant to the product due to mutations in the flea. If you're interested in eliminating fleas in your home, there is a great flea trap that will clean a whole room of fleas. They can be obtained from the Weston Company at www.wsthm.com or at www.myfleatrap.com. They are simple to use and do a great job. They will definitely prove or disprove the presence of fleas in your home.

Fly Strike

Fly strike is a term meant to explain the infestation of maggots in animal wounds. Normally there is considerable discharge of fluid around the lesion. When the lesion is cleaned, you will notice white maggots coming out of the lesion. They should all be removed and the wound cleaned with soap and water. If hydrogen peroxide is available, wash it out several times with the hydrogen peroxide. Since the maggots tend to get between the muscles, take your time cleaning. If you happen to have a Waterpik®, you can use it to get the maggots out rather easily. After getting the wound cleaned, you should treat it.

Treatment:

Clean and apply ointment to the area. Clean the lesion daily and reapply the topical ointment. Triple antibiotic ointments are available in grocery stores and pharmacies. Normally the strike is in an area that a bandage cannot be applied, but do your best and leave it open to heal in what is called third intention healing. Continue to treat with the ointment until it is healed. Remember that feed stores and tractor stores have good horse topical ointments that may be of benefit in cases such as this. You can obtain penicillin from feed and tractor stores, but they may have other antibiotics also. If other antibiotics happen to be available, you can use 10 mg per pound of body weight twice daily for fourteen days.

Hair Loss:
Fleas and Demodex

Hair loss has many causes, but the most common are mites and flea allergy dermatitis. I would say that flea allergy and Demodex are the top two causes of hair loss. A flea allergy takes time to occur since the flea injects a protein that combines with a portion of a protein in the body to form a heptane. This is the allergy producer, but it takes time for this to occur—and it is the result of not treating the animal for fleas. The hair loss starts just forward of the tail on the back of the dog and moves forward down the back and most cases are about midway up the lumbar region of the back of the animal. It can involve much more of the body. Demodex can be anywhere on the body and there can be widespread hair loss—or coin-sized lesions at any location on the body.

Scabies can also be the cause of hair loss. In cats, it seems to get a really good start on the margins of the ears but can be all over the face. We have seen some horrendous infections of the skin with this disease. Scabies can be transmitted to you and your family members—you will start scratching at little red dots. Unfortunately, this is a frequently misdiagnosed condition, so if you take someone to see the family physician who is doing a lot of scratching, explain that your pet has scabies. Another cause of hair loss can be chewing at the skin or self-trauma. Skin loss can also result from scraping along a highway after being hit by a car. These phenomena have been described earlier in this book—except for being hit by a car.

Treatment:

Check the proper category for the specific parasite and the correct treatments. For skin scraping along the highway, the wound should be treated as a burn. Sometimes more than skin is missing—so is muscle and bone. It is better to let your veterinarian do this one for you. However, you can medicate with triple antibiotic ointment and bandage the area. You can obtain some excellent horse topical medications from feed or tractor stores. You must change the bandage frequently and apply new bandages at least every other day. You cannot treat the wounds once and forget them. The wounds must be treated every day and it is best to treat the wounds two times daily. Bandages are hard to put—and keep—on pets. Be patient and do the best you can with what you have from where you are. I think the best thing to do with highway burn and tissue loss it to get to your doctor of veterinary medicine as soon as possible.

Hot Spots

Hot spots on a dog are the result of not treating it properly for fleas. The lesion is normally moist with matted hair and is quite painful to the dog. Prevention of this syndrome is preferred and very simple—just treat for fleas on a monthly schedule. Once the hot spot occurs, it is necessary to treat the wound or wounds.

Treatment:

Clip the hair on and around the lesion. The lesion may be so painful that your dog will not cooperate with you. After clipping the hair, wash the lesion. Repeat frequently during the treatment. Washing the lesion is good treatment for the hot spot. Any mild soap will do well. After washing and drying, apply 1 percent hydrocortisone cream to the lesion. This is a moist ointment and the animal may get onto furniture—so be aware that it could make a mess. You many need to keep the pet confined for a short period of time. The lesion should be cleaned and ointment reapplied at least twice daily until the skin lesion or lesions are healed.

External Parasites:
Ear Mites, Scabies, Lice

I lump these together because you can easily treat them all at one time with one over-the-counter drug—without much fuss. As I mentioned earlier, fleas are also an external parasite, but the same over-the-counter drug I recommend for these conditions will not treat fleas. Likewise, Demodex, or the so-called red mange (due to the red color caused by Demodex mites) is treated differently, but with the same over-the-counter drug. It will be covered under Demodex or red mange. My grocery store sells syringes and mm or cc measuring cup in one package. These products for measuring over-the-counter drug by cc or ML (the same unit just different names) are available over-the-counter.

The product—Ivermectin—is available at feed and tractor stores. We have used this compound on thousands of dogs and cats at our facility with no issues whatsoever. Even dogs that have tested positive for heartworms have had no issues. This drug is good and safe if proper dosage is used. If you happen to overdose a little, it is not a problem. Our road officers give this drug to every animal that comes into our facility; they give the dosage indicated by weight in the chart below. It will also treat hookworms and roundworms and will prevent heart worms if given a single dose per month. This is a great over-the-counter drug for your use. *It is recommended that it not be used in puppies younger than six weeks old.* However, I have done so in puppies that have scabies mites and have repeated the dose several times with no effect to the animal, but with great effect on the scabies.

Young kittens have a wide margin of safety for this product—it takes massive overdosing to cause issues in kittens. Feel safe to use it in young and old cats without reservation—but do not overdose. *The drug can be given orally or by injecting under the skin.* If it is injected under the skin, some animals feel a slight pain—more for cats—and it lasts for a few minutes at the injection site. However, it is far less painful than any disease that they may have that is being treated or prevented. This product is safe for pregnant animals as well. Ivermectin has proven to be rather effective for the treatment of ear mites by giving the drug orally according to weight and dose in the chart below or putting a small amount directly into the ear. When I put it into the ear, I normally dilute the Ivermectin with water fifty-fifty, but many do not do this. Dogs and cats will scratch at the ears infected with ear mites and cause damage—so treat the ears. We have used this drug to treat rabbit ear mites. The dose is given by weight (see chart) one week apart and the gunk on the ears just falls off all by itself. Do *not* attempt to remove it—leave it alone and it will come off all by itself after treatment. We have used Ivermectin in guinea pigs, rats, mice, ferrets, and other animals that come into our shelter and never had an issue. The chart lists dosage by weight. The dose is good for any animal—as long as the dose used is from the chart below. Mice and other small animals are less than a pound so you have to figure their dose. *Collie breeds with gene mutations are more sensitive to this drug so it is recommend that Collies and other related breeds not be treated with this drug.* There is no way that you can look at a Collie and tell whether it has the gene mutation, but you can have it checked if you feel that it is important. If you want the gene checked, talk to your veterinarian.

Treatment:

Follow the dose per the weight of your pet. This chart is only good if you purchase 1 percent Ivermectin. It is a large-animal product for cows, pigs, or sheep. For your information, Ivermectin is not officially approved for use in dogs and cats.

1 Percent Ivermectin Dosing Chart
(Weight Divided by 80 = Dose in CCs)

Weight Pounds	Dose ccs	Weight Pounds	Dose ccs	Weight Pounds	Dose ccs	Weight Pounds	Dose ccs
1	0.01	21	0.26	41	0.51	61	0.76
2	0.02	22	0.27	42	0.52	62	0.77
3	0.03	23	0.28	43	0.53	63	0.78
4	0.05	24	0.30	44	0.55	64	0.80
5	0.06	25	0.31	45	0.56	65	0.81
6	0.07	26	0.32	46	0.57	66	0.82
7	0.08	27	0.33	47	0.58	67	0.83
8	0.10	28	0.35	48	0.60	68	0.85
9	0.11	29	0.36	49	0.61	69	0.86
10	0.12	30	0.37	50	0.62	70	0.87
11	0.13	31	0.38	51	0.63	71	0.88
12	0.15	32	0.40	52	0.65	72	0.90
13	0.16	33	0.41	53	0.66	73	0.91
14	0.17	34	0.42	54	0.67	74	0.92
15	0.18	35	0.43	55	0.68	75	0.93
16	0.20	36	0.45	56	0.70	76	0.95
17	0.21	37	0.46	57	0.71	77	0.96
18	0.22	38	0.47	58	0.72	78	0.97
19	0.23	39	0.49	59	0.73	79	0.98
20	0.25	40	0.50	60	0.75	80	1.00

Weight Pounds	Dose ccs
81	1.01
82	1.02
83	1.03
84	1.05
85	1.06
86	1.07
87	1.08
88	1.10
89	1.11
90	1.12
91	1.13
92	1.15
93	1.16
94	1.17
95	1.18
96	1.20
97	1.21
98	1.22
99	1.23
100	1.25

Ringworm
Fungal Infections

So-called ringworm is not worms, and it does not have to be in the shape of a ring. In fact, most of the time, it is not. It comes in all shapes for sure. It is caused by the organism *Microsporum canis*. If the fungal infection is not caused by this organism, the fungal infection is not ringworm. There are many types of fungus that can attack your pet, but the so-called ringworm is the most common found. This condition is more common in cats than in dogs, but it may be a close race. This lesion causes hair loss and normally looks like a dry lesion. If you look closely, the hair is just barely seen on the skin as little dots of hair. There normally is no scratching at the lesion, but there can be. It is difficult to look at a lesion and determine whether it is a fungal infection.

An aid to seeing ringworm—specifically *Microsporum canis*—is to use a black light. Turn out the lights and shine the black light on the lesion. If you see granny apple green, you may have ringworm or a fungal infection. It can be difficult to identify the color since there are other things that glow under the black light. I find that the stubble or really short hairs appear green. If you happen to be wrong, it is not a big deal since the medicine will not harm the patient and is easy to apply.

Another aid might be if members of the family have skin lesions or if it has been diagnosed by your physicians in family members. The lesion can look just like a small Demodex lesion, so you could be wrong. To be sure, you have to take your pet to the doctor for a good diagnosis. You can treat it and if your diagnosis is correct , the lesion will resolve. If it does not heal, schedule an appointment with your veterinarian. The lesions between the toes may also be fungal infections and can be treated with the same compound. There may be multiple lesions on the cat—and on longhaired cats, it is hard to find and treat.

Treatment:

There are several fungal creams and powders, but I like Tinactin® cream. It comes in a small tube and is available in grocery stores and pharmacies. If you happen to be in the military, it is also in commissaries, the PX, and BX. It is easy to use; all you need to do is moist the lesion with the cream.

Sebaceous Gland Cysts

Sebaceous glands are glands of the skin that secrete oils through a duct to the skin surface. A cyst occurs when a sebaceous gland duct becomes plugged. The gland continues to produce the oils, but it cannot be excreted so there is an enlargement at the site of the plugged duct. The duct and gland start to get larger due to the continual secretion of the oil within the duct. Gland cysts will vary in size and may become large or stay small. Quite often, they get to a specific size and stay about that size for long periods of time. Others continue to grow and get bigger. They normally contain gray oils if ruptured or cut. They can be treated with over-the-counter items. Treatment is aided if you have a syringe and some hydrogen peroxide. You can purchase a bottle of hydrogen peroxide at any grocery store, pharmacy or Walmart.

Treatment:

If the gland is ruptured, traumatized, or cut, you can squeeze the gland to get as much of the oil out of the duct and gland as possible. Fill the syringe with hydrogen peroxide and flush the gland with the hydrogen peroxide. Continue to do so until the hydrogen peroxide stops bubbling and it runs as clear as it comes out of the bottle. Leave the gland alone and it will heal quite well and normally does not reoccur.

Skin Wounds

Skin wounds have all kinds of causes—from fights to gunshot wounds to cars and others. All wounds need to be cleaned with soap and water and the hair—as best as possible—needs to be clipped around the wound. If you have hydrogen peroxide available, it is a good idea to use it on the wounds. Animals that have wounds are in pain and if you hurt them more, they will bite. It is a really good idea if possible to muzzle or tie the mouth shut before getting vigorous with any trauma area on a dog or cat. After getting the wound clean, it is ready to be treated. You can get topical medications at pharmacies, grocery stores, and feed and tractor stores. Some horse topical medications are excellent for these types of wounds. I like to use nonstick bandages such as telfa pads next to the wound so that, when you change the bandage, you do not pull off the healing portion of the wound with the bandage.

Treatment:

Topical over-the-counter medications that you have purchased should be applied and the wound bandaged. Some areas of dogs and cats are not easy to bandage and it may be hard to keep the bandage on the wound so one has to be inventive. Bandages must be changed frequently. Some antibiotics are available at feed and tractor stores, mainly injectable penicillin (in small dogs, one to one and a half ccs, medium dogs, two ccs, and large dogs, three ccs). Small cats get one half cc and medium and large cats get one to two ccs. All of these doses must be injected under the skin (subcutaneously) and repeated twice daily for seven to ten days or until healed.

Chapter 5

The Eyes Have It

They certainly give strange names to diseases.

—*Plato*

Eyes are a very important organ for any living creature and need our proper care to sustain sight. The unfortunate thing about eyes is that they can be destroyed so quickly that one may never understand how it could happen so easily and quickly. Proper care and treatment of the eyes is perhaps more essential than treatment to other, less sensitive organs of the body. Here we will focus on keeping and maintaining good eyesight in our pets.

Cherry Eye

Cherry eye is a condition of the third eyelid in which the third eyelid gland has become displaced and is over the lower eyelid, making it visible in the corner of the eye by the nose. The condition almost always requires surgery to correct. Cherry eye can occur in one or both eyes and treatment with ointments and liquids normally does not help this condition. On occasion, the gland enlargement may be due to an infection of the gland, which can and has caused swelling of the gland enough to cause cherry eye. However, this seems to be a rather rare occurrence event for this particular gland. When taking your pet to see your pet's doctor, you should ask the doctor what procedure will be done to correct the cherry eye. There are two procedures: removing the gland or surgically moving the gland into the proper position in the third eyelid.

Treatment:

The removal of the gland can produce a dry eye or eyes in the future since the gland normally produces about 50 percent of the tear film or moisture for the eye. Your pet's doctor may offer the removal of the gland for fewer dollars. If so, be aware of the possibility of dry eye or eyes in the future. Of course, the treatment of choice is to surgically return the gland to the bottom of the third eye lid just as it was before it became displaced. Just be aware that when the gland is surgically replaced, it may become displaced or prolapsed again.

Bulging or Proptosis Out of the Eye Socket

Displacement of an eye forward or proptosis of an eye is normally due to some type of head trauma, resulting in the eye bulging out of its socket. Some breeds already have bulging eyes so they are more prone to proptosis than other breeds are. Bulging of the eye out of the socket can be partial or complete. If the eye is out and dangling, the eyesight is lost and the animal will most likely have to have the eye removed completely. If the eye is out in only a small way, it can easily be pushed back into place. The determination of the removal of an eye depends on the conditions of the traumatized eye. Removing the eye will be necessary if the optic nerve is severed, the eye globe is ruptured, the eye is infected, or the eye is dried.

Treatment:

The treatment by the owner is to keep the eye as moist as possible with water or eye ointments, if available, and go to your pet's doctor or emergency hospital as fast as possible.

Eye and Nasal Discharge in Cats

There are numerous causes of eye and nasal discharge in cats. For example, an upper respiratory condition or multiple types of infectious conditions can occur that complicate the medication choice for these conditions. Nonetheless, the eye and nasal discharge often has been successfully dried up using over-the-counter compounds that are available from pharmacies, such as CVS and Walgreens.

Treatment:

Different pharmacies have their own brands, but the generic name is chlorpheniramine maleate. The name at Walgreens is Wal-finate®; at CVS, you can find Chlor-Trimeton® and the CVS brand is Allergy Relief®. All of these compounds are chlorpheniramine maleate and they come as 4 mg tablets. Give ¼ of a tablet to your cat once daily or, if necessary, twice daily. Never give more than one complete tablet [4 mg] in twelve hours. The dosing may need to continue for ten to fourteen days. Continue the medication until the cat is dry and then continue for at least two additional days. Sometimes dipping the ¼ of a tablet into tuna fish juice may help the medicine go down.

Foreign Body behind the Third Eyelid

Sometimes a foreign body, such as a small piece of grass, a weed, sand, or other items will manage to get between the third eyelid and the eyeball. These objects cause considerable pain and damage to the eye—especially the cornea—and can develop into an ulcer. Foreign bodies behind the third eyelid will cause ulcers on the cornea next to the nose. The trick is to pull the third eyelid forward and look behind to see if there is an object present. If there is, you can remove it.

Treatment:

Unfortunately, you are limited as to what you can do since the condition is often so painful that the animal will not stand for anyone messing with its eye. Your veterinarian can use a topical anesthetic that will almost immediately stop the pain and allow for an exam behind the third eyelid for removal of foreign bodies. You can flush the eye with copious amounts of water and sometimes the foreign body will flush out. Other times, the foreign body can become lodged in the tissue of the third eyelid and any effort at flushing the eye will not remove the foreign body from behind the third eyelid. You will need your friendly veterinarian's help with this condition. Remember that eyes can be very delicate and there are no second chances with the eyes. Have it looked at quickly—do not wait to have the eye examined.

Inward Rolling of the Eyelid Margin (Entropion)

Entropion is the inward rolling of the eyelid margin—the areas of the eyelids where the eyelashes are located. Unfortunately, this condition is common in many species. Rolling in of the eyelids can be very subtle and hardly noticeable in some mild cases, especially if the dog or cat is excitable. When there is inward rolling of the eyelids, there is a constant tearing from the corner of the eye by the nose. This causes discoloration of the hair below the rolled-in eyelid. Normally, this type of inward rolling of the eyelids necessitates surgery to stop the constant tearing from staining the hair under the eye. This condition can cause eye sores such as corneal ulcers or be the cause of infections of the eye and cause considerable pain to the pet. Inward rolling of the eyelid (entropion) can be congenital or present from birth, or it can be a spastic condition of the eye muscles causing the eye to be drawn back into the eye socket, perhaps scar tissues from a wound or it may occur subsequent to a particular positioning of the eye. Congenital entropion is the most frequently type of entropion in dogs, but is not as common in cats. However, it does occur. It is not uncommon for conformational type entropion to affect both eyes. The upper eyelid is not as often involved in this condition; the lower eyelid is frequently involved with rolling of the eyelid onto the eyeball.

Spastic entropion occurs due to spasms of the eye muscles—mainly the so-called orbicularis oculi muscle—because of painful eye conditions such as ulcers on the cornea, infections of the outer eye, or infections of the iris. Topical treatment often can correct the entropion due to the elimination of pain. Complete medical corrections and treatment of the eyes—to be sure that the entropion is not due to pain resulting in spastic entropion—is recommended before undergoing entropion surgery. Regardless of the type of entropion, treatment before surgery will be helpful as well as diagnostic in confirming the need for surgery.

There is a duct that runs from the eye into the nose that is called the lacrimal nasal duct. The job of the lacrimal nasal duct is to transport the eye fluids into the nose. This is what causes you to have to blow your nose a lot when you cry. If this duct becomes plugged or blocked, the tears or eye film can no longer be discharged through the duct and will run over the eyelid and down the face.

Treatment:

The inward rolling condition of the eyelids that are conformational or present due to scars must be corrected surgically. The spastic entropion may only require keeping the eye moist with a tear product such as GenTeal which is available at CVS, Walgreens pharmacies, and Walmart stores. This may require eye medicine that your veterinarian can provide. The blocked lacrimal nasal duct normally requires medicine from your pet's doctor.

What to Do with Hair in the Eyes of Dogs and Cats

Unfortunately, hair in the eyes of many animals is a source for eye ulcers, infections, and pain. Many breeds have hair in the eye and many are seen in shelters with matted hair in the eyes, resulting in foreign body (hair) stimulated tear production.

Treatment:

Clip the hair around the eyes and keep it short. It is important that the hair be properly cut since cut hair in the eyes is worse than the mass of long hair due to the sharp, tough end of a cut hair. The hair needs to be cut routinely to prevent eye damage. Help a dog see. Keep the hair around the eyes cut properly.

Eye Infections

Your pet's eyes are so important that it is essential you take your pet to see its doctor. However, if you will not under any circumstances do so, then there may be an alternative available for you. However, be aware that pets can have what is called a melting ulcer of the cornea. Regardless of what you do, the eye may—and often does—become much worse in just a couple days. It may cause a hole in the cornea. Eye issues are very, very important and need to be taken care of rapidly.

Treatment:

Feed stores have a product called Terramycin ophthalmic ointment; call to see if the store by you has the product. If they do, you can put ¼ inch of the Terramycin in the infected eye a minimum of four times per day. If you can obtain a small EDTA blood tube [it has a purple top rubber stopper in the tube] and put sterile water into the tube, you can use three to four drops about ten minutes before you put the Terramycin in the eye, this will often prevent melting ulcers. *It is far better to let your veterinarian do your pet's eyes for you since you could harm your pet's eyes with improper treatment.*

A Single Ruptured Blood Vessel on the White of the Eye (Sclera)

There are many causes of a single ruptured blood vessel and it is impossible to know what or how the bleeding has occurred. However, it is a phenomenon that has created lots of concern and lots of questions. To date, many of these types of events have been observed in dogs, cats, and people. There has never been—in my experience—any further trauma or occurrence. The bleeding raises lots of concerns—mainly due to the fact that it is so readily seen—though there is little need for concern.

Treatment:

Given time, the bleeding of the single blood vessel will resolve without treatment. All that is necessary is a bit of time. It may look bad for a period, but it will resolve on its own.

Chapter 6:
Skin Challenges to be Conquered

I will prepare and someday my chance will come.
—*Abraham Lincoln*

Skin conditions seem to spring up overnight and wreak havoc on the skin. Skin conditions can quickly become—or cause—superficial or systemic syndromes that may include simple hair loss, self-mutilation by excessive scratching, or biting and eating of one's self. Therefore, careful observation and quick intervention into skin conditions will prevent advanced superficial skin or early skin penetration conditions from becoming a major issue, resulting in unnecessary expenses and poor health for your pet.

Sores around the Ears of Cats

Often there are lesions caused by the cat around its ears. The sores may be in front or behind the ear or lower on the neck. Ear mites cause the cat to scratch at the ear. Rather than scratching the ear, cats seem to scratch in areas close to the ear. Sometimes it is so bad that muscles can be seen in the areas where the cat has been scratching.

Treatment:

Treatment is quite simple; the ears need to be cleaned and Ivermectin should be put into the ear. The wounds will start to heal because the cat will stop scratching at the ears. Ear cleaning was explained in chapter one page 1 "cleaning ears" after the ears are clean you can put some Ivermectin in the ears to treat any ear mites that are present.

Miliary Dermatitis of Cats or Feels like Fine Sand on the Skin

Miliary refers to small seeds (2 mm in size) or small sand-like objects. These granules on the skin can be found and easily felt on the neck and head of cats that have been badly infested with fleas. This is a sure sign that the cat needs to be treated for fleas.

Treatment:

To treat the fleas apply Advantage to the back of the neck just back of the head so the cat cannot lick the medication.

Mosquito Bite Hypersensitivity in Cats

Mosquito bite hypersensitivity is not a common finding among cats, but many readers of this book may have seen this syndrome and not known what the cat had. The hypersensitivity may be mild or severe. The occurrence of the condition is most obvious during the mosquito seasons. It can cause the cat to scratch a lot. Normally the sores can become rather raw and red, appearing as an infection of the head and ears. Foot pads may be darker than usual, particularly on the edges of the pads. The pads may be swollen and painful or may lose some skin. The bridge of the nose may be swollen and the end of the nose may be swollen. Swelling at the tip of the nose seems to be more noticeable when looking from the side. The cat may also have swollen lymph glands. The signs of mosquito hypersensitivity are similar to other skin conditions, which makes mosquito hypersensitivity difficult for the untrained eye to detect and therefore a need for your cat to visit the cat's doctor. Mosquito bite hypersensitivity can cause permanent scarring of the skin.

Treatment:

It is always best to keep the cat away from possible insect bites by keeping the cat indoors. Even indoors, a mosquito might be able to get into the house and bite. Open sores can be treated with antibiotic ointments applied to the sensitive lesions. Warning: Many human mosquito repellents, such as Deet®, may be toxic to your cat. If ointments are used on your cat, be aware that the ointments can stain furniture.

Excessive Hair Shedding of Dogs

Hair shedding is normal in dogs and cats. Some animals shed more hair in the spring and fall. In fact, some animals shed much more than other animals do. Some pets seem to shed hair all year. The good news is that there are no developments of areas of exposed skin due to hair loss.

Treatment:

There is no treatment for this condition. Excessive hair shedding is a normal, healthy condition. Daily grooming will help to keep the hair loss away from furniture and other areas in the house. A good balanced diet is necessary. Supplementing the diet with Omega-3 fatty acids may be of great benefit for the skin of the pet that has excessive hair shedding.

Hair Loss between the Eyes and Ears of Cats

It is normal to have hair loss between the eyes and ears of cats. The condition is more readily visible on shorthaired cats than on long haired cats. Some cats will have almost no hair in this area between the eyes and ears, but others will have very little missing. This is not a disease and is quite normal for cats.

Treatment:

None—this is normal in domestic cats.

Hunting Season and Working Dog Foot Pad Trauma

Many hunters like to use dogs during hunting season for game bird pointing, retrieval of game, and other trained hunting skills. At the start of hunting season, the dogs have been idle most of the year. When hunting season arrives, it is out to the woods or fields to hunt with the dogs. The feet of the dogs have become tender due to lack of activity and the foot pads can be completely removed on the first day of hunting due to the dogs running through such things as dried sunflowers or other weed patches that can cause the dog to become lame. The trauma received by the removal of the foot pads puts hunting with the dog on hold while the dog's feet heal.

Treatment:

If at all possible, the dogs should be taken out often to keep the foot pads in condition for the hunting season. Obtain Tuf-Foot and apply to the pads; it will help to make the pad more callused and tough enough to withstand the rigors of the hunting surge. If the dogs have not been out frequently and the feet have become tender, it is advisable to start applying the Tuf-Foot about four to five weeks before hunting. When the foot pads become worn off, the feet can be treated with any antibiotic ointment obtainable at grocery stores and pharmacies and the feet can be bandaged. Rest is then in order to allow for healing and re-growth of the tissues on the foot pads. Tuf-Foot is available online at http://www.tuffoot.com . Tuf-Foot is packaged in a small container that is easy to use—just soak a cotton ball with Tuf-Foot and apply it to the feet. Tuf-Foot dries rather quickly. However, be aware that it might get on rugs or furniture if you are not careful when applying the compound to the feet.

Lack of Pigment on the Nose or Nasal Vitiligo

Lack of pigment or nasal vitiligo of the nose allows the nose of a dog to be exposed to sunlight, resulting in sunburn and possible cancer due to the sun. Many dogs have this condition and there is a need to protect the nose from overexposure to sunlight. The sunburn can be very painful and discomforting. Nasal cancer can be disfiguring.

Treatment:

Sunblock can be used on the dog's nose. Some have had the nose tattooed to prevent excessive sun exposure.

What Shampoo Should I Use?

If your dog has skin issues, many different types of shampoos will help. These products are normally dispensed by your pet's doctor. This discussion will focus on bathing non-diseased skin. In all likelihood, there are hundreds of fine shampoos that are okay for pets. My recommendation is the result of asking clients what shampoo they used on their pets. The question was directed to owners whose pets smelled good, had soft, fluffy hair, and looked really nice.

Treatment:

I asked, "What have you been using to bathe your dog?" The answer was almost always Johnson's Baby Shampoo—so this is the recommended product. It does a great job. As a result of the many, many responses to the question, the author has used the same shampoo daily for forty years and still has hair.

My Dog Has Dry Skin. What Can I Do?

Most dogs have glands that secrete oils onto the skin and hair. Some dogs have an issue with dry skin and what to do for dry skin is a commonly asked question. Bathing a dog too often can cause dry skin. Many dogs have dry skin that can be treated with moisture therapy products.

Treatment:

Once the dogs have been bathed, fill a bucket of warm water and pour a capful of Alpha Keri into the bucket and pour it onto the pet. Alpha Keri is a product for moisture therapy and can be purchased online or at drugstores.

Chapter 7:

Easy to Prevent, but often Hard and Expensive to Treat

Cheers to a new year and another chance to get it right
—*Oprah Winfrey*

It has been said that an ounce of prevention is worth a pound of cure. This is certainly true for the health of our pets and the protection of our pocketbooks. In this chapter, we will focus on how to keep our pets free of some rather nasty diseases and conditions. Your pet does not want to experience any of them, but with the knowledge of how to prevent the syndromes, they can be averted. They will live happily ever after.

You can prevent a pet from becoming ill from many diseases and syndromes simply by being alert and knowing and doing the right things at the right time to save the health and wellbeing of your pet. This chapter will point out several of the simple conditions that you can easily prevent.

Rocky Mountain Spotted Fever

Rocky Mountain spotted fever is a tick-transmitted disease that is cause by a rickettsia, which is an organism that is smaller than bacteria, but larger than a virus. Rocky Mountain spotted fever is like so many diseases that may be more prevalent in some areas than in other areas. This was truer in the past than it is today because of the transient nature of the people in the United States and world. This disease is considered to be a very important disease in humans. The disease can be very debilitating and cause lethargy, dehydration, and little spots of hemorrhage (so-called petechial) and other signs that the pet's doctor will see if you fail to prevent it. Rocky Mountain spotted fever can be a life-or-death disease for your pets.

Treatment:

Prevention is your role; this syndrome can easily be prevented by a good monthly tick control program. If at all possible, avoid known tick-infested areas with your pet. Use a good product such as Advantix II [formally Advantix], which is an improved tick and flea product. If you're a hunter and go out frequently with your dogs in areas known for Rocky Mountain spotted fever, a check with your veterinarian would be of potential benefit. Your veterinarian can dispense Doxycycline for a weekly preventive treatment that will also help prevent the disease. Remember that no prevention is 100 percent assured. When returning home, comb out your dog's coat and check closely for ticks. You can remove ticks by hand, but you should use disposable gloves when performing this process because ticks carry diseases.

Salmon Poisoning (Pacific Northwest)

This disease has a higher prevalence of occurrence from San Francisco to Alaska due to the availability of raw salmon, trout, or Pacific giant salamanders that contain metacercariae of a rickettsia-infected fluke. The organism invades the small intestinal tract and lymph nodes. Signs of the disease include diarrhea, vomiting, nasal and ocular discharge, and fever. This can be another life-threatening disease for your pet if the animal becomes infected. Salmon poisoning requires a trip to your pet's doctor—and the sooner, the better because it will most likely have to be hospitalized. Animals will normally die in five to ten days if not treated. With the transient population, even though the Pacific Northwest is the primary area, this disease may be seen elsewhere in the county.

Treatment:

Prevention is the key for this disease. Do not to allow your pet to eat any raw salmon, trout, or Pacific salamanders. Owners must be alert for potential ingestions of products that will cause salmon poisoning.

Antifreeze in Cabin Toilets in Mountain or Ski Areas

Antifreeze in toilet water is a potential killer of dogs because their kidneys can be badly damaged by antifreeze in cabin toilets. The family arrives at the cabin and starts to move and settle into the cabin. However, if the toilet seat is up and the dog drinks the water, it can obtain ethylene glycol poisoning. Not knowing that the dog has drunk the water out of the toilet, time is lost until the dog becomes sick and is taken to the dog's doctor. It may be too late to save its life, depending on how observant the owner is and how quickly the dog is taken to the veterinarian. Sadly, this author has seen this avoidable scenario repeated.

Treatment:

This is a preventive treatment. Turn off the water to the toilet, flush the toilet, and make sure that all the water is out of the tank and toilet bowl. Or keep the toilet seat down and place weights on the seat—some dogs will still manage to open the toilet seat enough to get their head into the toilet bowl when the toilet seat is left down. Many people mistakenly think that they have kept the dog from getting to the toilet bowl. If you see the dog drink the water from the toilet that has antifreeze in it, you can induce vomiting with hydrogen peroxide, a very strong salt solution, or syrup of ipecac. These procedures are so simple, but have been heartbreaking for many folks. It is hard to believe that it happens, but it does.

Grape or Raisin Toxicity

It may be hard to believe, but grapes and raisins will cause kidney failure in dogs. To date, no other species are known to be sensitive to grapes or raisins. The toxic dose is very small—in the range of .03 to .13 ounces per pound of body weight of grapes and .15 to .43 ounces per pound of body weight for raisins. Normally, dogs will vomit within twenty-four hours of ingesting raisins or grapes. If the syndrome continues, it will end with the death of the dog. The signs are quite similar to those of ethylene glycol toxicity.

Treatment:

Prevention is the primary key to this syndrome. However, if you see a dog eat grapes or raisins, you can induce vomiting with hydrogen peroxide, a concentrated salt solution, or ipecac syrup. If ipecac is used, give .5 to 1 CC per pound of body weight up to a maximum of 15 CC. A heavy concentrated salt solution can be made quickly by heating water with lots of salt. The salt will dissolve—use the resulting solution to induce vomiting. Call a poison control center or your veterinarian as soon as possible.

Feeding Raw Eggs

Feeding raw eggs to animals is considered a no-no because the raw white contains avidin, which binds to biotin, resulting in a B vitamin deficiency. The binding of avidin to biotin is so strong that even if B vitamins are supplemented, it will not overcome the deficiency cause by the avidin. Cooking the egg will destroy the avidin.

Treatment:

Prevention is quite simple. Cook any eggs fed to animals—or do not feed uncooked eggs to your pet.

Chocolate Poisoning

When an owner leaves out a box of chocolates, dogs can eat a lot of it. A little does not harm, but a bunch does. The chocolate contains theobromine and caffeine. The caffeine is quickly metabolized and excreted, but the theobromine is not secreted as fast and causes toxicity. Early signs are vomiting and loose stools. It normally takes only one to two ounces to be a problem.

Treatment:

Prevention is the treatment of choice. Keep chocolates away from pets. If the package of chocolates is out, it should be closed. Remember that dogs will get up on furniture or tables to get to food when they are not being watched. If the consumption of the chocolate is observed, then vomiting needs to be induced with hydrogen peroxide, a concentrated salt solution, or syrup of ipecac [if ipecac is used, give .5 to 1 CC per pound of body weight up to a maximum of 15 CC]. A heavy concentrated salt solution can be made quickly by heating water with lots of salt. The salt will dissolve—use the resulting solution to induce vomiting. Call a poison control center or your veterinarian as soon as possible.

Lyme Disease

Lyme disease is spread by Ixodes ticks. They are the major carriers of the disease and when they attach to pets, they suck blood and inject the bacteria that cause the disease. The signs of Lyme disease are reminiscent of many other syndromes, but the diagnosis is easy for the pet's doctor due to the available testing equipment. The disease tends to primarily infect dogs, but rarely cats. The disease is more prevalent in the Midwest, Northeast, Southeast, and South Central United States. The disease is most prevalent where there are larger numbers of deer and small rodents. If there are no deer in an area, the incidence of Lyme disease is very low or nonexistent.

Treatment:

The best treatment of this disease is prevention. A Lyme disease vaccine would be recommended in areas where the disease is most prevalent. However, one needs to remember the transient movement of pets from one area to another that can transform non-tick areas into infected areas in short order because ticks lay thousands of eggs very quickly. Avoid areas that are known to be heavily infested with ticks and treat the dog as directed by flea and tick preventive compounds such as Advantix II, which kills tick, fleas, flea eggs, flea larvae, and mosquitoes with a single treatment. When returning from any outdoor areas with your pet, comb and check the pet for ticks. Examine the dog carefully and remove any ticks using a disposable glove. Dips for ticks are also capable of helping to prevent Lyme disease. If your pet is suspected of having contacted the disease, it is highly recommended to take your pet to see the doctor as soon as possible because the disease gets worse with time.

Problems with Homemade Cat Foods

Taurine is an essential amino acid in the diet of cats. Cats need to metabolize bile acids and cannot do so in the absence of taurine in the diet. This condition is self-induced by homemade diets that don't include taurine. In our current age of commercial diets, this essential amino acid has been added to prevent taurine deficiency. Some dogs will develop and manifest the signs of taurine deficiency. The most prone are American cocker spaniels and some giant breeds [Newfoundland]. On occasion, other breeds may also develop taurine deficiency. Taurine deficiency normally results in retinal degeneration and heart failure. Fortunately, heart failure can be partially—and in some cases—fully reversed with taurine supplementation. Since taurine is not essential for dogs, many dog foods are not normally supplemented with taurine. In modern diets, this condition is not seen as much as it once was, but it still can be an issue.

Treatment:

Prevention is important with this disease. It can easily be prevented by feeding normal commercial cat and dog foods because they have been supplemented to prevent taurine deficiency. For the diehard homemade diet folks, taurine can be purchased from health food stores—and normally at reasonable prices. There are no known side effects of taurine.

Tick Paralysis

If you happen to live in an area where there are large numbers of ticks, it is a good idea to use a flea-tick preventive such as Advantix II every month to prevent tick paralysis and other diseases. Tick paralysis is caused by female Ixodes ticks and several other ticks that secrete salivary neurotoxins, causing paralysis of pets. If an owner takes the dog for a walk in the woods or in a pasture, the dog might pick up a few ticks. The signs are gradual; unsteadiness and weakness are seen in the hind limbs and, if left alone, become worse as the paralysis progresses. Animals can be down within three days; the limbs become limp or flaccid and the dog does not move. Tick paralysis can—and has—resulted in death of pets. If it is recognized in its early stages and not in final death throes, you can easily treat the pet.

Treatment:

Be diligent in the use of flea-tick products and look for ticks between the shoulder blades and up and down the back of your pet. If found, pull any ticks off. It is best when removing ticks to use disposable gloves and wash your hands really well when finished because ticks can be infected with diseases. Regardless of the condition of the pet, a good search for the ticks should be accomplished. Once the ticks are removed, the pet will recover from the paralysis—in my experience—within a few hours. A tick type dip is very beneficial for the treatment of this condition as well as Advantix or Advantix II.

Plants in and around the House that are Poisonous to Pets

There are, of course, so many plants that it is impossible to list every plant that has the potential to harm your pets. So many households have plants around or in the house that can be dangerous to pets, but we will focus on the more common ones found and ingested by pets. This list is not complete nor is any attempt made to make it complete. The top ten called into the Pet Poison Helpline are autumn crocus, azalea, cyclamen, Kalanchoe, lilies, oleander, dieffenbachia, daffodils, and lily of the valley(lilies are highly toxic to cats), sago palm, tulips, and hyacinths. If you see your pets eat any of these plants, you should call your veterinarian or one of the poison help centers. The number for the Pet Poison Helpline is 1-800-213-6680 and the number for the ASPCA is 1-888-426-4435. The following is a grouping of the plants and types of signs that they may or may not be produced if eaten. Poisoning depends on the plant, the type of toxin in the plant, and the amount of the plant consumed. Some of the plants will cause multiple system problems, such as intestinal, heart, or central nervous system signs. Those that have more than one body system effect will be listed more than once. For greater details on each plant, call a poison help center.

Unfortunately, depending on the dose of plant toxin that is consumed, the signs are not as neatly identifiable as the following list makes them out to be. Do not hang your hat on one or two signs, but know what plants you have in or around the house. If you have to take your pet in for eating a plant, take some of the plant with you to the veterinarian.

Plants that are known to cause vomiting, diarrhea, drooling, and depression include Sago palm, azalea, rhododendron, oleander, castor bean, cyclamen, yew, amaryllis, autumn crocus, chrysanthemum,

English ivy, peach lily (Mauna Loa peace lily), Kalanchoe, marijuana, and dieffenbachia.

Plants that affect the heart include Kalanchoe, oleander, daffodils, lily of the valley, azalea, rhododendron, and yew.

Plants that cause central nervous system signs, including convulsions, seizures, and coma include yew, tulips, narcissus bulbs, castor bean, marijuana, and possibly lily of the valley.

Plants that can cause liver failure or kidney damage include the sago palm and autumn crocus.

Treatment:

The best treatment is prevention. Either do not have the plants around or keep your pet away from your toxic plants. Treatment for any of the above is best handled by your pet's doctor because the treatments are quite complicated and intense if the animal is to survive. The signs from any of the plants can be mimicked for each of the plants listed and can be similar to non-plant toxins. Time is very important in order to give the pet the best possible chance for making it through the ordeal of ingesting poisonous plants.

Poison Help Centers

There are numerous poison control centers. We present two here for quick reference in the event that such a need arises for your pet. The ASPCA Poison Center telephone number is 1-888-426-4435; the telephone call is free, but the consultation is about $65. Another poison center is the Pet Poison Helpline (1-800-213-6680); again, the telephone call is free, but the consultation is about $35. Each has specific and different things that they would like for you to have available when you call. The most important thing for you to do is keep calm, cool, and collected. Take a deep breath and count to ten. You must be able to communicate with the person on the other end of the telephone.

ASPCA: Have the species, breed, age, sex, weight, and number of animals involved in the event. Be able to explain the signs exhibited by the animal. If possible, any information about the agent that your pet has consumed helps a lot—or if you can, have the container available with its label. Finally, always consult your veterinarian or the ASPCA poison center for directions on how and when to use any emergency aid.

Pet Poison Helpline: Remove your pet from the area and check to make sure your pet is safe, is breathing, and is acting normally (depending on the poison, acting normally may be impossible). Do not give any home antidotes. Do not give hydrogen peroxide without first talking to your veterinarian or poison helpline. Do not use hydrogen peroxide in cats—it does not stimulate cats to vomiting. Do not stimulate vomiting without talking to your veterinarian or poison helpline. If veterinary attention is necessary, take your pet, the poison, and label on the poison with you to your veterinarian immediately. Another poison center that takes calls about dogs, cats, iguanas, goats, guinea pigs, horses, spiders, and fish is the Washington State Poison Center. The Washington State Poison Center telephone number is 1-800-222-1222; you may call this number to tell about emergency poisoning, ask questions about poisons, or ask questions about poison prevention. The Washington State Poison has Mr. Yuk stickers that you can purchase to put on items in your home if you happen to have young children. They charge $30 for calls about pets. For more information, call the poison center of your choice.

Household Hazards

Numerous household hazards can be detrimental to your pet's health. Ingestion of house hold hazardous compounds and liquids most often results in the need for an emergency telephone call to the poison center or your veterinarian for treatment information or guidance of what to do at the scene of the ingestion..

Alcohols: Ethanol, methanol, and isopropanol are the most common around a household. Ethanol is in most varieties of alcoholic beverages. Methanol is commonly found in windshield washer fluids. Isopropanol is in rubbing alcohols and alcohol-based flea spays. Signs normally start between twenty and thirty minutes after consumption.

Chlorine bleach: This is found in household cleaners, clothes bleach, and some pool chemicals. Since pets have been contaminated by chewing on plastic items that have had bleach in them, it is important to keep them away from pets. If splashed into an eye, the eye can be badly damaged and need to be flushed.

Corrosives, acids, and alkaline products: Acids include anti-rust compounds, toilet bowel cleaners, gun-cleaning compounds, automotive batteries, and swimming pool cleaning agents. Alkaline agents include drain openers, automatic dishwasher detergents, toilet bowl cleaners, radiator cleaning agents, pool algaecides, and shock agents. These products can cause burns on tissues, skin, feet, and internal organs.

Alkaline batteries: Remote controls, hearing aids, toys, watches, computers, and calculators can result in burns and can penetrate some tissues.

Cationic detergents: Algaecides, germicides (including dryer softener sheets), and others can cause ulcers or burns on mouth tissues, esophagus, stomach, and other delicate internal tissues. Signs include excessive salvation, swollen tongue, vomiting, and abdominal discomfort.

Detergents, soaps, and shampoos: These are the least corrosive and toxic, but they can be very bad for a pet's health. Items include mild detergents, soaps, and shampoos with anionic or non-ionic ingredients. Grooming cats may develop rather severe signs of toxicity.

Avocado: Has been a cause of heart damage in dogs; Guatemalan varieties are most toxic.

Many more products around the house can be devastating to a pet; some can even cause death rather quickly. More on these and other poisons can be found in the *Merck Veterinary Manual, Tenth Edition, 2010*: p 2553–2592.

Treatment:

Keep cleaning and other compounds properly stored and properly dispose of empty containers. If a pet does consume a toxic compound, contact your veterinarian or a poison control center as soon as possible for guidance and treatment. In the case of toxins, an ounce of prevention is worth more than a pound of treatment.

Rabies

Rabies is a deadly disease that can be prevented. Unfortunately, many people ignore the proper immunizations for their pets and many animals have been infected with rabies. Rabies immunizations are required in most states within the United States for dogs and cats. The first immunization is normally good for only one year. This is due to the fact that there is no way to know the extent of the animal's immune system. Furthermore, the first immunization sanitizes the immune system of the animal to provide a much stronger immune response at the time that the second rabies immunization is given. To provide the best protection for the pet, a second immunization is required one year later. In most states, the second immunization is good for three years. Cats are more likely not to be immunized—they are ten times more likely to contract the disease than dogs are. Dog owners tend to have their dogs immunized, but owners of cats do not.

Treatment:

Have your pets immunized to protect the pet, your family, friends, and visitors.

Distemper

Distemper is a viral disease that affects dogs and other animals. The infection attacks the nervous system, the intestines, the respiratory system, and essentially all systems of the body. It is closely related to measles and foreign animal diseases, such as rinderpest. Raccoons and skunks bring the distemper virus into local neighborhoods at night. If feeding bowls are left out overnight, they will eat out of these bowls and leave saliva infected with the distemper virus. Even after many years of pet immunizations, the disease continues to be present and causes infections in dogs. All ages are susceptible to the disease. The disease has an incubation period of seven to twenty days. The virus does not last long outside of the body and can be easily disinfected with phenolic or quaternary ammonium compounds.

Treatment:

The best approach to this disease is prevention. Immunize your pet. Modified live vaccines protect for three years. Current guidelines are to vaccinate dogs at six to eight weeks of age—with repeat vaccinations every three to four weeks until sixteen weeks of age. All dogs should receive a booster at one year of age and then every three years. Vaccines are available at feed stores and low-cost immunizations can be obtained at organizations, such as Luv My Pet.

Chapter 8:

Nutrition and Other Digestive Tract Occurrences

An intellectual is a man who takes more words to tell more than he knows.

—Dwight D. Eisenhower

The digestive tract alpha and omega is so diverse, long, and specialized that one has to marvel at all the activity that occurs in such a short tube of the body. Each station along the tract is different, but functions so well that we think nothing of it until it goes haywire and then it is a mess. In this chapter, we will be stopping at different stations along the elemental canal to examine phenomena that are of interest to us to help our pets be our buddies and friends for a long time.

My Pet is not Eating. What Should I do?

This is a frequently asked question and there are many very bad things that cause pets to stop eating. You need to take your pet to see the pet's doctor because there is normally some systemic disease process that is stopping your pet from eating.

Treatment:

Take your pet to see its doctor. It is far better for the veterinarian to tell you that there is nothing to worry about than hesitating and having the delay cause your pet to die. Be safe and take your pet to see the doctor.

Should I Feed Table Scraps to My Pet?

No, you should not. Will you? Yes, you will. The issue with feeding scraps to your pet is that it can cause your dog or cat to not have a proper diet. You care about your pet or you would not be reading this book. Where I work, we see dogs and cats that have been on the loose. If they are lucky, they have been able to scrounge table scraps from garbage cans. These animals are never healthy; you are treating your dog as though it is a stray by feeding what is left over. Now why mistreat your pet? I know you're going to tell me that you were feeding table scraps to your pet before I was born. You may be right about that, but when you take your pet to see the veterinarian because it is sick, remember that I said not to feed garbage to your pets. Feeding bones is bad because bones can get stuck in the roof of the mouth, puncture the stomach or intestines, or result in constipation. You don't see what veterinarians see. There is no such thing as a free pet—so take good care of the critter.

Treatment:

Obtain a good cat or dog diet and feed the dog or cat correctly. Be a buddy to your pet—not a miser.

Feeding Omega-3 Fatty Acids

Omega-3 fatty acids have been found to be beneficial to pets as well as people. Omega-3 fatty acids aid the skin. There are certain diseases that they also help cure—and might even help prevent. At our clinic, a lady was so impressed with the results of feeding Omega-3 fatty acids to her hypothyroid dog that she told me to be sure to tell you about it. Fatty acids are good for itching syndromes, (pruritic) inflammation diseases, allergies, feline eosinophilic granuloma, and crusting disease. It also aids healing of yeast infections of the skin.

Treatment:

Approximately 20 percent of dogs and 50 percent of cats with allergic itching (pruritus) will show some improvement. Large doses may cause weight gain or diarrhea—a good rule of thumb would be about 500 mg two times daily. Omega-3 fatty acids in fish oil are the best source and can be purchased in grocery stores, vitamin shops, Costco, B.J.'s, pharmacies, and Walmart. The main fish oils are eicosapentanoic acid (EPA) and docohexanoic acid (DHA). Salmon, herring, sardines, and mackerel will also provide EPA and DHA (Omega-3) to pets.

Yellow Tooth Syndrome

The use of tetracycline medications in young animals—normally less than six months of age—causes yellow teeth. The drug becomes accidently dispensed and—due to the young age of the animal—the adult teeth are still developing. The yellow color of the tetracycline medicine becomes embedded in the enamel of the developing adult teeth and there is nothing that can be done to reverse this condition. The animal will have yellow teeth for the rest of its life.

Treatment:

Know that tetracycline and second—and third-generation tetracycline drugs (Doxycycline) will cause yellow teeth in young animals. If someone dispenses tetracycline-like drugs to your pet when it is younger than six months, call their attention to the fact that they have done so and ask to have the drug changed to another antibiotic.

Aging Cats and Dogs by their Teeth

Aging any animal by their teeth is an approximation and is by no means accurate. However, it may work as a ballpark determination for an animal's age. Different animals do not necessarily have their teeth come in at the same time as other animals do. They also may have considerable variation as to the development with age. In bygone years, dog and cat teeth were pretty much ignored. However, in these millennia, many pet owners have the teeth cleaned and provide routine daily and/or weekly brushings of their pet's teeth, which alters older age determinations. Furthermore, there are now items on the market to aid in helping to keep teeth clean and aid breath smells. Nonetheless, sometimes determining an age is important. This chart will help you obtain a ballpark age for your pet and other dogs and cats:

ESTIMATED AGE	CAT'S TEETH	DOG'S TEETH
2–4 Weeks	Deciduous (baby) incisors coming in	No noticeable tooth growth
3–4 Weeks	Deciduous (baby) canines coming in	Deciduous (baby) canines coming in
4–6 Weeks	Deciduous (baby) premolars coming in on lower jaw	Deciduous (baby) incisors and premolars coming in
2 Months	All deciduous (baby) teeth are in. Normally all deciduous (baby) teeth are close together until 2 months of age. They spread at 2 months.	All deciduous (baby) teeth are in. Normally all deciduous (baby) teeth are close together until 2 months of age. They spread at 2 months.
3.5–4 Months	Permanent incisors coming in	No noticeable permanent tooth growth
4–5 Months	Permanent canines, premolars, and molars coming in	Permanent incisors coming in; some growth of premolars and molars
5–7 Months	All permanent teeth are in by 6 months	Permanent canines, premolars, and molars coming in; all teeth in by 7 months
1 Year	Teeth white and clean	Teeth white and clean
1–2 Years	Teeth may appear dull with some build-up (yellowing) on back teeth	Teeth may appear dull with some tartar build-up on back teeth
3–5 Years	Teeth show more tartar build-up on most teeth and some tooth wear	Teeth show more tartar build-up on most teeth and some tooth wear
5–10 Years	Teeth show increased wear and disease with some pigment on gums	Teeth show increased wear and disease
10–15 Years	Teeth are worn and show heavy build-up; some teeth may be missing	Teeth are worn and show heavy tartar build-up; perhaps teeth missing

Vocal Cords Blocking the Wind Pipe (Trachea)

This condition occurs infrequently, but when it does, it horrifies owners and they are dumbfounded as to what to do or what the cause is. The problem is that the vocal folds become unattached and—due to a slight vacuum that is created in the trachea—the vocal folds are pulled out into the trachea, causing a considerable blockage of the trachea or windpipe and making it very hard for the pet to breathe. The signs in dogs include the dog putting its head down toward the ground and between the front legs; the front legs are spread wide apart in a sawhorse stance. The dog tries hard to breathe, but cannot get enough air and the tongue, mucus membranes, or gums turn pale or blue. This is an emergency and it can kill the pet. This condition can be—and often is—intermittent. When it stops, the owner thinks it is over—but then it occurs again and it might kill the pet.

Treatment:

This condition has no over-the-counter treatment or prevention that an owner can perform. It is presented due to the many clients that have experienced this with their pet and have grave concerns and are very stressed for their pet. The owner needs to get the dog to the pet's doctor as soon as possible. The treatment is surgical removal of the vocal folds, which reduces the volume and sound of the dog's bark.

The Danger of Sewing Needles

This frequent condition is caused by leaving sewing needles out so that the cat can get to them. The curiosity of cats will help them find the needle. For some odd reason, they attempt to swallow them—or carry them off—and they get stuck in the back of the throat. One has to surmise that the condition is very, very painful and it can be prevented.

Treatment:

Unfortunately, the cat will not let you stick your fingers into its mouth—you will get bitten. This requires a trip to see your cat's doctor. The best thing to do is to be very conscious of the fact that you have a cat—and if you sew, you *must* put the needles away so the cat cannot get to them.

Sewing Thread—a Deadly Hazard for Cats

Sewing thread is a killer of cats. Cats will get at any item—thread, small necklaces, or rubber bands—and swallow it. The thread or small thread-like items will then start to go through the intestines. The problem is that only a portion of the thread will go through the intestine. The intestines make all kinds of bends and kinks and the thread starts to cut on the bends and kinks of the intestines—and essentially becomes a saw. The thread will cut completely through the wall of the intestines. When the bends and kinks of the intestines are cut open by the thread, the contents of the intestines get into the abdominal cavity. The cat will be sliced up and down the intestinal tract—and get a bad infection in its abdomen.

Treatment:

The treatment is simple. It is called prevention. Just keep thread and thread-like items put away so that cats cannot get to them. Some costume jewelry is like thread and one often finds such items on bathroom sinks or cabinets. Cats can get to the items and swallow them. Just do not leave such items lying around. Remember that the cat's life you save could be your own cat's life.

A Special Note about Tapeworms

It has been noted by the pathologist at the Bronson Animal Disease Diagnostic Laboratory in Kissimmee, Florida, that animals which have experienced anesthesia death have lung infections that appear to be linked to extra heavy infestations of tapeworms in the intestines.

Though this finding is a clinical evaluation and not a scientific study, it would be in keeping with good parasite control programs to have your pet treated for tapeworms at least four to six weeks before having surgery to allow any lung infection—if it is in fact caused by the tapeworms—to heal. The challenge is getting a diagnosis because many fecal flotation examinations do not show an active infestation unless a small part (a proglottid) of the tapeworm has broken open to allow eggs to be seen in the fecal exam. The most common signs are white to light yellow wiggling worms on the feces of your pet. These are proglottids that have broken off the tapeworm. Tapeworm infestations—depending on the species—are not normally detrimental to pet's health. New products on the market, such as the Bayer's Profender, will treat most tapeworms. If you happen to be getting this product from your veterinarian, your pet may not need any further treatments for internal parasites. However, there are some species of tapeworms that Profender will not eliminate.

Treatment:

To treat tapeworms, you can you use three products that are sold at Petco, Pet Smart, tractor stores, and feed stores. The products you need are either praziquantel or a Pyrantel-praziquantel combination. Follow the directions on the labels of the purchased product. Panacur may be used to treat tapeworms. If Panacur is used, see the Panacur dosing table by weights for dogs and cats. The chart can be found on page 84. You can purchase Panacur from feed and tractor stores as a liquid horse or cow wormer, but make sure that you purchase 100 mg per CC Panacur.

Using Panacur for Treatment of Hookworms, Roundworms, Whipworms, and Tapeworms

The following chart provides the necessary doses of Panacur for treating tapeworms. Panacur can be purchased at feed and tractor stores. The product will be either a cow [bovine] or horse [equine] product. Panacur comes as a paste or a liquid. Liquid Panacur is easier to handle and dose so it is recommended that you purchase 100 mg per CC liquid Panacur. The container is rather large and will last a long time. The expiration date will be posted on the bottle—try to get the bottle with the expiration date as far into the future as possible. Panacur is a great product and will treat hookworms, roundworms, whipworms, and tapeworms.

Treatment:

Use liquid 100 mg per CC Panacur solution. Shake well and withdraw the dose indicated in the chart for the weight of your dog or cat. Give the indicated dose by weight once daily for three days. *Do not overdose.* Use a CC or ML syringe or measuring devise to measure the treatment dose.

100 mg/CC PANACUR [FENBENDAZOLE] DOSING CHART

(WEIGHT times X 25 divided by 100 = Dose in CC's)

Weight Pounds	Dose ccs	Weight Pounds	Dose ccs	Weight Pounds	Dose ccs	Weight Pounds	Dose ccs
1	0.25	21	5.25	41	10.25	61	15.25
2	0.50	22	5.50	42	10.50	62	15.50
3	0.75	23	5.75	43	10.75	63	15.75
4	1.0	24	6.0	44	11.0	64	16.0
5	1.25	25	6.25	45	11.25	65	16.25
6	1.50	26	6.50	46	11.50	66	16.50
7	1.75	27	6.75	47	11.75	67	16.75
8	2.0	28	7.0	48	12.0	68	17.0
9	2.25	29	7.25	49	12.25	69	17.25
10	2.50	30	7.50	50	12.50	70	17.50
11	2.75	31	7.75	51	12.75	71	17.75
12	3.00	32	8.0	52	13.0	72	18.0
13	3.25	33	8.25	53	13.25	73	18.25
14	3.50	34	8.50	54	13.50	74	18.50
15	3.75	35	8.75	55	13.75	75	18.75
16	4.00	36	9.0	56	14.00	76	19.0
17	4.25	37	9.25	57	14.25	77	19.25
18	4.50	38	9.50	58	14.50	78	19.50
19	4.75	39	9.75	59	14.75	79	19.75
20	5.00	40	10.0	60	15.0	80	20.0
						81	20.25
						82	20.50
						83	20.75
						84	21.0
						85	21.25
						86	21.50
						87	21.75
						88	22.0
						89	22.25
						90	22.50
						91	22.75
						92	23.0
						93	23.25
						94	23.50
						95	23.75
						96	24.00
						97	24.25
						98	24.50
						99	24.75
						100	25.0

Coccidia Treatment with Marquis (Ponazuril)

Marquis is a prescription drug for horses. If you happen to have horses, you may have some of this compound around. Those who are not horse folks might be able to get your veterinarian to write a prescription for this compound. Marquis can be purchased online with a prescription at www.agri-med.com . It is a paste and can be purchased as 127 grams or 150 mgs/gm in a 120 mg volume tube. Treatment with this compound is much simpler than with Sulmet or Albon (Sulfadimethoxine), which requires several days of treatment. The Marquis compound is diluted with tap water 1 CC of Marquis to 1 CC of water or 10 CC of Marquis to 10 CC of tap water essentially one to one. The dose is given .1 CC per pound of body weight or 1 CC for 10 pounds (see chart below). Dose once and then repeat the same dose in ten days and again in two weeks. Marquis is very simple and a very effective treatment.

MARQUIS (PONAZURIL) DOSING CHART

(DOSE IS .1 CC PER POUND OF BODY WEIGHT)

Weight Pounds	Dose ccs	Weight Pounds	Dose ccs	Weight Pounds	Dose ccs	Weight Pounds	Dose ccs	Weight Pounds	Dose ccs
1	0.1	21	2.1	41	4.1	61	6.1	81	8.1
2	0.2	22	2.2	42	4.2	62	6.2	82	8.1
3	0.3	23	2.3	43	4.3	63	6.3	83	8.3
4	0.4	24	2.4	44	4.4	64	6.4	84	8.4
5	0.5	25	2.5	45	4.5	65	6.5	85	8.5
6	0.6	26	2.6	46	4.6	66	6.6	86	8.6
7	0.7	27	2.7	47	4.7	67	6.7	87	8.7
8	0.8	28	2.8	48	4.8	68	6.8	88	8.8
9	0.9	29	2.9	49	4.9	69	6.9	89	8.9
10	1.0	30	3.0	50	5.0	70	7.0	90	9.0
11	1.1	31	3.1	51	5.1	71	7.1	91	9.1
12	1.2	32	3.2	52	5.2	72	7.2	92	9.2
13	1.3	33	3.3	53	5.3	73	7.3	93	9.3
14	1.4	34	3.4	54	5.4	74	7.4	94	9.4
15	1.5	35	3.5	55	5.5	75	7.5	95	9.5
16	1.6	36	3.6	56	5.6	76	7.6	96	9.6
17	1.7	37	3.7	57	5.7	77	7.7	97	9.7
18	1.8	38	3.8	58	5.8	78	7.8	98	9.8
19	1.9	39	3.9	59	5.9	79	7.9	99	9.9
20	2.0	40	4.0	60	6.0	80	8.0	100	10.0

Chapter 9:

Trauma and Other Uh-Oh Occurrences

Now this is not the end. It is not even the beginning of the end. But, it is perhaps, the end of the beginning.
—Sir Winston Churchill

Uh-oh—that was not supposed to happen, but it did. How could it have been avoided and how can we prevent it from occurring again? Confucius is supposed to have said, "I hear and I forget. I see and I remember. I do and I understand." We will focus on being prepared to see and react appropriately for the health and comfort of our pets without panicking.

Sunstroke or Excessive Body Temperature

Sunstroke can be a hidden, incognito condition taking place before your very eyes. Unless you're aware that it happens, you may lose your pet due to trying to be buddies with your dog and taking your dog for a walk. As you walk, the body temperature becomes highly elevated. We will discuss two major causes of elevations of body temperature that can and do result in death of the pet. The most innocent condition is to take a dark-colored dog for a walk on a hot day with temperatures above 90 degrees and low humidity. Dogs do not sweat. They lose body heat by panting; as the dog walks on the sidewalk or road, they add to the heat of the day and the dog will start to have an elevated temperature. A small walk of one to one and a half miles out and then back has killed some dogs. The signs of elevated body temperature are not obvious. The mouth, gums, or mucus membranes may turn bright red. Some folks have described the color of the mouth appearing as red as a tomato or a cherry. This is about the only notable sign that is not always present. If the dog is not cooled down quickly, its temperature can quickly get to 107 degrees—or higher. If the body temperature raises this much, the dog is doomed because there is no coming back from such high temperatures. The author has seen dogs with this exact scenario that have had temperatures so high that they could not be measured on a thermometer. The other syndrome is also very preventable—and is the most common cause of killing dogs by causing body temperatures to rise rapidly and fatally. Leaving a dog in a car on a hot day with the windows up is a disaster just waiting to happen. Just don't do it.

Treatment:

The best treatment is prevention. If the temperature is 90 degrees or higher, do not walk the dog at the peak of the day's temperature. Wait until it is cooler in the day. If you do walk the dog, check the color of the mouth frequently, go for short distances, and go quickly back to a cool place. If you notice the dog's mouth getting red, get the dog in a pool as soon as possible and let the dog rest there. If you happen to be by a lake, get the dog in the cool water. It is important to act fast and be patient with the dog. Let it get cooled down before finishing your walk. As for leaving a dog in a car with the windows up on a hot day, this is a bad, dumb thing to do. However, it happens unbelievably often. If you are going somewhere and you know you cannot take the dog inside, do not take the dog with you. In Orlando, folks go to Disney and leave dogs in their cars all afternoon, which is so regrettable. Make sure that it does not happen to you or your pets. Be wise—not sad.

Lip Swelling Due to Angioneurotic Edema or Angioedema of Dogs

Angioneurotic edema is a condition noticed when the lips (flues) of a dog become enlarged and the swelling appears to be an abscess. It often occurs rather rapidly—sometimes overnight—and is noticed in the morning as the night before the dog was completely normal. For the unknowing, it is not uncommon for the swelling to be mistaken for an abscess. The lesion looks just like a large abscess but when it is stabbed with a surgical blade with the expectation of draining exudate from the swelling there is no draining exudate present. Unfortunately it is often stabbed again and again there is no draining of exudate. Perhaps it is stabbed several times expecting to drain an exudate from the swelling all to no avail because it is an edematous swelling not an abscess. It is not caused by an infectious agent; but by cellular and intracellular edema causing the enlargement of the lips. In appearance, it is a rather large swelling of the lip—normally on one side of the mouth. For owners, it is always an alarming syndrome and a cause of great concern. The cause is surmised to be due to an insect for which I cannot vouch, but the author has seen many such cases of Angioneurotic edema.

Treatment:

Leave it alone—it will go away all by itself. No treatment is necessary.

Hospitalization Due to Dog Bites

Dog bite hospitalization jumped 86 percent in 16 years in the United States, according to government analysis. In December 2010, the Department of Health and Human Services Agency for Research and Quality announced that that the number of people hospitalized because of dog bite-related injuries had increased from 5,100 to 9,500 in 2008. The most often bitten were children under ten years of age and senior citizens. Males were seen at emergency departments more often than women were. However, there was no sex difference between male and female hospitalizations. In the United States, in 2008 there were an average of 866 emergency department visits and 26 hospitalizations every day of the year. An estimated 4.7 million people are bitten by dogs annually. The main reason for hospitalization is due to infections from bites of extremities or wounds on the head, neck, and trunk. Young children are the most likely to be hospitalized. Additionally, there were four times as many dog bite-emergency department visits and three times as many hospitalizations in rural areas as there was in urban areas. More information can be obtained from the *American Veterinary Medical Association Journal* [JAVMA] Feb 1, 2011, Vol 238:3: pp 274.

Treatment:

Selection of a good pet is a serious business when young children and seniors are in the household. Care should be taken to assure the safekeeping of these folks in the absence of good supervision. Large dogs are more capable of mauling younger children than small dogs are. If you have a dog that tends to bite and you have small children, you should reconsider the pet's position in the family relative to the safety of the children and/or seniors in the household.

Mumps

Mumps is a common disease for people, but it is rare in dogs. Dogs sometimes catch the disease from young children. It will affect dogs of all ages and there is no sex preference. The signs are normally only an elevated temperature and lethargy and loss of appetite. In addition, the parotid salivary glands are often enlarged. The parotid glands are located at the angle of the mandible or the lower jaw under the ears on both sides of the dog's head. The enlarged glands could be mistaken for cancer; however, other glands may not be involved. Mumps only spreads from acutely infected people to dogs and not from dogs to people. This is not what would be considered a normal disease for dogs. [Tilly, L.P. & F.W.K. Smith Jr. *Blackwell's Five-Minute Veterinary Consult: Canine & Feline*, 2007:4: pp 902-903]

Treatment:

Normally, there is no need for treatment of the dog. The noticeable lethargy will stop in five to ten days. If the dog is ill beyond the normal ten days, then it would be reasonable to have the dog checked for hydration and electrolyte deficiencies at the dog's favorite doctor's office.

Rattlesnake Bites

Dog often get bitten by rattlesnakes—and, in some areas, rattlesnakes can be quite large. In others, they are rather small and the problem that the dog has is dependent upon the amount of venom injected by the snake. Rattlesnakes cause necrosis—tissues dying rapidly—causing swelling, discoloration, and pain due to the toxin injected. Rattlesnakes can be found throughout the United States. Though rattlesnakes are rare in some areas, they can be in large numbers in other areas. It is important to be watchful for rattlesnakes in certain areas. In fact, in some areas of the country, they have had rattlesnake drives to help depopulate the large populations of rattlesnakes.

Treatment:

A vaccine is available that helps protect dogs from the effects of rattlesnake bites. It is available at your veterinarian's clinic or hospital (Red Rock Biologics Rattlesnake Vaccines). Your veterinarian can help you decide if the vaccine is the right protection for your dog. The vaccine works by stimulating an animal's immunity to defend against potentially harmful agents. The rattlesnake vaccine is intended to help create an immunity that will protect your dog against rattlesnake venom. There is not much an owner can do once the dog has been bitten by a rattlesnake. Even though the dog is vaccinated against rattlesnake venom, the dog should be evaluated by a veterinarian. Your veterinarian can determine if the dog will need further treatment.

Lying to Your Veterinarian

I know that this topic sounds stupid, but you would be surprised at the large number of people who do lie to their veterinarian. Lying makes no sense at all, but it happens. The main reason for lying is embarrassment about the condition that is present in the pet because it may appear as neglect—and sometimes it is. It seems odd because the reason that the person is present is to aid the health of their pet; correct information about the condition is essential to help provide the pet with the best care possible. Of course there are fees involved—why lie? This author has actually had clients say "Next time, I will not lie to you."

Treatment:

Do not lie to your veterinarian—they want to help you and your pet. Considering the pet's symptoms, it is usually obvious that the person is lying. Remember that honesty is the best policy.

Foreign Bodies in the Nose

Foreign bodies in and up the nose seem to be more common in hunting dogs because they are out in weeds and sticks. It is common for dried weeds to break off and manage their way to the nose of dogs. The normal complaint upon presentation to a veterinarian is that the dog seems to be doing a lot of sneezing. Tops of cattails, parts of dried sunflowers, and other foreign bodies have been found in dog noses.

Treatment:

If there seems to be a lot of sneezing, look up the nose. If a foreign body is seen, attempt to remove the object. Many have been quite easy to reach. However, some items need the help of your dog's doctor.

Reverse Sneeze

Reverse sneezing is a normal, protective, repetitive respiratory reflex that aids in removing irritants from the nasopharynx, which is the area above the soft pallet that communicates with the nose and windpipe. The sneeze is often the result of some mild irritant. It is often sudden and repeated. Dogs often hold their heads up—or pull them back with the mouth closed. If observed, closely the lips or flues may be noted to be sucked into the inside of the mouth.

Treatment:

This is normal reflex and in no treatment is usually necessary unless it is consistent and persistent. Due to the nature of the complicated reverse sneeze, it may require a visit to your veterinarian.

Kennel Cough

Kennel cough is very common in dogs—and it is easily transmitted in crowds of dogs at kenneling facilities, dog parks, and other areas wherever dogs gather. The signs are coughing and the intensity and persistence seems to be more pronounced in the evening when the temperatures start to cool. It is best to let the cough be productive because coughing moves materials out of the lungs. Once a dog gets kennel cough, it is best to allow the dog's doctor to provide the necessary medicines. However, there are some things that you can do.

Treatment:

A vaccine is available in two versions: one for up the nose and one for injection under the skin. Both vaccines protect against kennel cough. The nose kennel cough (Bordetella) is called mucosal immunity and tends to provide immunity at the site of infection. It provides good protection. The injection is also protective, but the nasal immunization is considered to be somewhat better. The vaccine needs to be repeated in six months to be able to maintain good protection from the disease. If the dog is coughing at night or just before you go to bed, you can give Robitussin DM, which will help suppress the cough. Give large dogs two teaspoons, medium dogs one teaspoon, and small dogs half a teaspoon. For puppies, give a half-teaspoon of infant drops. Each size and dose can be repeated every four hours if needed. During the day, you want the cough to be productive so do not suppress the cough. Your dog's veterinarian can best provide medicines for this condition if your pet happens to get this disease.

Grass Awns

Grass awns are powerful, burrowing seeds that get onto pets when they come in contact with the seeds of awn-producing grasses. They burrow into the skin and migrate to almost any position on the body. They either cause draining tracts or thoracic or abdominal cavity infections. The draining tract is a challenge to treat—with a mad search to find the grass awn that is causing the draining tract. However, it is such a challenge that it may never be located and the tract will continue to drain. The abdominal or thorax infections are potential killers. If they become completely filled with exudates from the infection, it is overwhelming for the pet and causes death.

Treatment:

Treatment is a prevention and avoidance program. Whenever a pet gets into tall grasses that have awns or suspected to have grass awns, it is important that the dog be inspected for the presence of grass awns. Quickly remove them. Be alert for any outdoor areas that contain tall grasses with awns. If identified, go around the grass because the problems will be very difficult to treat—and costly. After a day outside, inspect the dog for awns. Many folks have shaved the hair or cut the hair very short to find offending awns and prevent infections.

Umbilical Hernias

Small umbilical hernias are quite common. They are caused by a small hole in the body cavity—usually at the belly button area or the point at which the umbilicus was formerly attached. This small hole—normally about one to two millimeters in diameter—allows small amounts of fat to be expelled from the abdominal cavity just beneath the skin. The hernia may be movable or stationary. If movable, the hernia will disappear when the pet is on its back, but it will not disappear if it is not movable.

Treatment:

This is usually a cosmetic surgery that may or may not need to be done. The hernia normally establishes adhesions and a small hard pocket that prevents any movement of the contents in the hernia in or out of the abdominal cavity. If the hernia remains the same size, it is not necessary that the hernia be surgically repaired. If it starts to become larger, then it is necessary to have it repaired because other abdominal contents may be extruded. Cutting off normal circulation will potentially strangle the gut or other organs, requiring surgery to save your pet's life.

Head Tilt

Head tilt is a very common condition in dogs. It does occur in cats, but not anywhere near as commonly as in dogs. There are many causes of head tilt, but there is nothing that an owner can do with the condition due to the central nervous system. However, an owner can do a lot to prevent head tilt due to infected internal and external ear infections. One to the major causes of external ear infections is ear mites—and the failure to treat for ear mite infestation or keep the ears clean. The procedure for clearing and treating ear mites has been previously described in Chapter I. Floppy eared dogs have the greatest problem with ear infections—mostly due to owner neglect. Look often and keep the ears cleaned. "If it is to be, it is up to me!" This means you—the owner.

Treatment:

Prevention of internal and external ear infections is the correct action. This is rather simple and cheap to complete. Keep the ears clean and make sure that the ears do not become infested with ear mites. If you happen to be using prescription Revolution or Advantage Multi, then as you treat for fleas, you will be treating for ear mites as well. Do not forget to inspect the ears frequently and keep the ears clean. Once infected, it is a job for your dog's doctor.

Pets and Yards Recently Sprayed with Chemicals

Many of us want a nice yard and we hire or self-treat our yards with bug killers and fertilizer to make the yard greener. Unfortunately, lots of folks let their pets out on the freshly sprayed or treated yards and the pet becomes contaminated with the compound that has just been applied. Letting a pet on a freshly treated yard amounts to contaminating your pet with whatever compound happened to be put on the yard—and it may affect the pet adversely or even kill it. Since most of the compounds that affect pets require a good diagnosis and quick treatments, getting your pet to your pet's doctor is paramount. Tell the doctor what was applied to the yard if at all possible.

Treatment:

Prevention is the best plan of attack. If you know that the yard has been treated, keep your pet off until it is known to be safe. That might be three to four hours—or perhaps an entire day. Whatever the case may be, the delay will save the pet's health as well as saving the pocketbook from unplanned expenditures for yard chemical poisoning.

Ear Medicine Causing Hypersensitivity to Drugs

Dogs often have ear infections that have been treated with medications being put into the ear. After a while, the skin of the ear canal may start to turn red. As the treatment continues, there may be inflammation, the ear may become even brighter, and the pain may become worse. When this occurs, the dog has developed a hypersensitivity to the medicine being used to treat the ear. The problem is not an infection, but an allergic response to the medicine.

Treatment:

All medications being used to treat the ear infection need to be stopped so there is time for the hypersensitivity reaction to heal. Be patient for up to fourteen days. Normally, when the hypersensitivity is overcome, the dog's ear infection is also healed. There are always exceptions to any treatment, but in most cases, you will be pleased that you stopped the medications.

Ruptured Intervertebral Discs

Ruptured intervertebral discs are an emergency that needs to be seen by your veterinarian as soon as possible. Delay may cripple your pet permanently—or leave them unable to control urination, defecation, or movement of the rear legs. Two major syndromes occur normally in smaller dogs, but large breeds may have the same issues. The first syndrome is a cervical disc rupture. The normal scenario is when the dog jumps off the couch, it yelps and walks backward as if trying to get away from something. It will normally have its head down. These classic signs indicate that a disc has ruptured and is putting pressure on the spinal cord. The next most common syndrome is for a lumbar (lower back region) disc to rupture so that the dog loses sensation or movement of the rear legs. It may have limited use of the rear legs and may dribble urine. The issue in the lumbar area is the same as the one described for the neck—its intervertebral disc has ruptured. Dorsal moves will put pressure on the spinal cord. If not corrected quickly, it will permanently damage the spinal cord. It is possible that the pressure is so great that nothing can be done to reverse the trauma in the neck or lumbar areas. The dorsal lumbar disc protrusion is often seen in dogs that have been hit by cars.

Treatment:

There is nothing that an owner can do other than get his or her pet to the veterinarian as soon as possible to allow quick surgery. The sooner surgery can be performed, the better. Normally, in the neck region, the disc involved will be removed as much as possible to eliminate pressure on the neck region spinal cord. In the lumbar regions, a dorsal laminectomy is performed.

Gunpowder and Dogs

Gunpowder and dogs are not a good combination. This is most often an issue for a weapons enthusiast that loads his or her own ammunition. If there is gunpowder out, it is possible for the dog to eat some of the powder. It frequently burns a hole in the stomach or intestines and causes loss of appetite, lethargy, weight loss, and peritonitis. If the gunpowder perforates the stomach or intestines, it is a death knell.

Treatment:

Make sure that the dog cannot—and does not—eat any gunpowder. Whatever it takes, keep the dog away from the gunpowder.

Separation Anxiety of Dogs

Many dogs with separation anxiety exhibit problematic behaviors, such as destructiveness, excessive barking or whining, excessive salivation, vomiting, pacing, self-injury, anorexia, and perhaps withdrawal or inactivity among others. This syndrome can be helped greatly with the aid of your pet's doctor and by working on behavior modification. We will limit this discussion on what you can do to help your dog overcome this syndrome by working on behavior modification. If it is of any comfort, know that an estimated 10 million dogs in the United States suffer from this syndrome in some form or fashion.

Treatment:

First we want to reemphasize that your pet's doctor can help you with separation anxiety—so do not think that you can do this all by yourself. You can start your behavior change by being positive and focusing on the positive behaviors of your pet. Affection can be emphasized; treats and toys can be used to reward positive behavior. You should ignore your dog if it greets you as you come home or exhibits other attention-seeking behavior. Make no big deal out of coming and going. Do not say good-bye, pet, or do any other thing that brings attention to the fact that you are about to leave. A good exercise is to act out leaving home—grab your car keys, put on your coat, sit down, read the newspaper, watch TV, or spend time just sitting. After a period of time, take your coat off and put it away. Do not give attention to your pet, and do not pet the dog or talk to the dog. You can grab your keys, walk away, and then return the keys. Or perform other acts that you normally do just before leaving home and then do not go. Work on teaching you pet to stay in a certain area that the dog feels comfortable in and perhaps spend time in the area. The idea is to get the dog to feel comfortable in the area so that the dog will remain in the area when you are away. Patience is the name of the game. It will not happen in a day or two—it will take time.

Open Draining Sore Under the Eye

This has fooled a lot of people into thinking that the lesion is caused by an eye infection, but they could not be more wrong. The cause of this condition is an abscessed tooth and the tooth most commonly involved is the so-called carnassial tooth.

Treatment:

To treat this condition, the tooth must be removed. This will require a trip to the veterinarian. The pet will have to be given anesthesia. The carnassial is one tooth, but it has three roots and can be really difficult to remove.

About the Author

Dr. Robert Ridgway graduated from Kansas State University College of Veterinary Medicine and completed a residency in Internal Medicine at the University of California, Davis. After graduating from veterinary college, he worked for a short period of time at a veterinary hospital in Topeka, Kansas. He entered the US Army Veterinary Corps where he became director of the Animal Medicine Division on Okinawa. He later completed a residency of comparative medicine at the Madigan Army Medical Center. He is a graduate of Officer Candidate School at Fort Sill, Oklahoma, and a graduate of the US Army Command and General Staff College. He was the treasurer of the District of Columbia Academy of Veterinary Medicine for fourteen years. He served as secretary-treasurer and president of the District of Columbia Veterinary Medical Association. He was the first US Army officer to be in charge of the Department of Defense Military Dog Veterinary Service at Lackland Air Force Base in San Antonio, Texas. He completed a master's of international management at the University of Maryland, University College. After retiring from the army, he worked at Covance Laboratories, Banfield Pet Hospital and is currently employed at Orange County Animal Services in Orlando, Florida. Dr. Ridgway is a diplomate in the American College of Preventive Medicine and a diplomate in the College of Laboratory Animal Medicine. Dr. Ridgway is married and has one daughter and one male cat.

Index

A
Abscessed tooth, 99
Acids, 72
Advantage, 40, 57
Advantage Multi, 96
Advantix, 40, 69
Advantix II, 63, 67, 68–69
Aerophagia, 20–21
Age, estimating, 78–79
Aggression, 14
    See also Biting
Alcohols, 72
Alkaline batteries, 72
Alkaline products, 72
Allergic itching, 77
Allergic reactions, 35–36
Alpha Keri, 61
Anal glands, impacted, 8
Angioneurotic edema, 89
Antibiotics, 48, 77
Antifreeze, 64–65
Artificial tears, 5
ASPCA Poison Center, 70–71
Aspirin, 9
Avocado poisoning, 73
Awns, grass, 94

B
Bad breath, 16, 19–20
Bald spots, 36, 37–38, 41–42, 58–59
    See also Fur
Balls, stuck in throat, 3–5
Barbering, 36
Batteries, alkaline, 72
Bayer's Profender, 82
Behavioral problems, 13–17
Benadryl, 7–8, 27–28
Biting, 9–10, 14, 89–90
Biting flies, 36–37
Black stools, 24, 29
Body temperature, excessive, 87–88
Bones, feeding of, 76
Bulging eye, 50

C
Cabin toilets, 64–65
Car trauma, 42, 97
Carnassial tooth, 99
Carnation canned milk, 20, 21
Cationic detergents, 72
Cats
    defecating on floors, 14

excessive grooming of, 36
eye and nasal discharge in, 51
hair loss of, 58–59
hairballs and, 21
homemade food and, 67–68
loose stools and, 23–24
miliary dermatitis of, 57
mosquito bite hypersensitivity in, 57–58
petting-induced aggression in, 14
rabies and, 7, 73
sewing needles and, 80–81
sewing thread and, 81
sores around the ears of, 56–57
urine spraying in, 14–15
Cervical disc rupture, 97–98
Cherry eye, 49–50
Chlorine bleach, 72
Chlorpheniramine maleate, 51
Chocolate poisoning, 66
Choking, 3–5
Coccidia, 22, 29, 30–31, 85–86
Collars, embedded, 6–7
Collies, 22, 30, 44
Congenital entropion, 52–53
Constipation, 20
Coprophagia, 16–17, 19
Corn oil, 39
Corneal ulcers, 51, 52–53, 54
Cornstarch, 11
Corrosives, 72
Cottage cheese and rice diet, 25
Coughing, 2–3, 93–94
Cysts, sebaceous gland, 47

D
Dandruff, 25
Defecating on floors, 13–14
Dehydration, 22, 29
Delivery complications, 2
Demodex, 37–38, 41–42, 43

Detergents, 72–73
Diarrhea, 22–25, 29, 39
Diet
bones, feeding of, 76
dull hair coat and, 38–39
high fiber, 21
meat-exclusive, 25–26
obesity, 6
omega-3 fatty acids and, 76–77
table scraps and, 76
taurine deficiency and, 67–68
vegetable diets, 12
See also Pet foods
Discharge, in cats, 51
Discs, ruptured, 97–98
Dishonesty, 92
Distemper, 74
Dogs
with ball in throat, 3–5
bite-related injuries from, 89–90
defecating in house, 13–14
difficulty breathing, 80
excessive hair shedding of, 58
foot pad trauma in, 59
lip swelling in, 89
separation anxiety and, 98–99
Dorsal laminectomy, 98
Doxycycline, 63, 77
Draining tracts, 94
Drug hypersensitivity, 96–97
Dry eyes, 5, 50
Dry skin, 60–61
Dull hair coat, 38–39

E
Ear mites, 1, 43–45, 56–57, 95–96
Ears
biting flies and, 36–37
cleaning of, 1–2
hair loss between, 58–59
infections of, 1–2, 95–96, 96–97

mites, 1, 43–45, 56–57, 95–96
    sores near, 56–57
Eating, refusal to, 75–76
Eggs, 39, 65–66
Elbow dysplasia, 9
Embedded collars, 6–7
Entropion, 52–53
Ethanol, 72
Ethylene glycol toxicity, 64, 65
Eyes
    bulging or displacement of, 50
    cherry eye, 49–50
    corneal ulcers, 51, 52–53, 54
    discharge in cats, 51
    dry eyes, 5, 50
    foreign body in, 51–52
    hair in, 53–54
    infections of, 52, 54
    inward rolling of eyelid, 52–53
    open draining sore under, 99
    ruptured blood vessel in, 54–55

F
Famotidine, 34
Feces-eating, 16–17, 19
Feeding. *See* Diet; Pet foods
Fish oil, 77
Flatulence, 20–21
Fleas, 39–40, 41–42, 57
Flies, biting, 36–37
Fly strike, 40–41
Food. *See* Diet; Pet foods
Foot pad trauma, 59
Fungal infections, 46–47
Fur
    dull hair coat, 38–39
    excessive shedding, 58
    hair loss, 36, 37–38, 41–42, 46, 58–59
    shampoos, 60

G
Gas, intestinal, 20–21
Gas-X, 21
GenTeal ophthalmic ointment, 5, 53
Gland cysts, 47
Grape toxicity, 65
Grass awns, 94
Grass eating, 34
Gums, 22, 29
Gunpowder, 98

H
Hair loss, 36, 37–38, 41–42, 46, 58–59
    See also Fur
Hair shedding, 58
Hairballs, 21
Halitosis, 16, 19–20
Head tilt, 95–96
Heartworms, 43
Heatstroke, 87–88
Heimlich maneuver, 4
Helplines, poison, 70–71
Hernias, umbilical, 95
Highway burn, 42
Hill's Science Diet, 11, 26
Hip dysplasia, 9
Honesty, 92
Hookworms, 22–23, 29–30, 43, 82–84
Hospitalization, dog bite, 89–90
Hot spots, 42–43
Housebreaking, 13–14
Household hazards, 71–73
Houseplants, 69–70
Hunting dogs, 59
Hydrogen peroxide, 16, 41, 47, 48, 65, 66, 71

I
Immunization reactions, 7–8
Immunizations, 7–8, 73–74, 91, 93–94
Imodium, 22–24
Impacted anal glands, 8
Induced vomiting, 64–65, 66, 71
Infections
    ear, 1–2, 95–96, 96–97
    eye, 52, 54
Intestinal parasites, 22–24, 29–33, 81–86
Ipecac syrup, 65, 66
Isopropanol, 72
Ivermectin, 30, 37–38, 43–45, 57

J
Johnson's Baby Shampoo, 60

K
Kennel cough, 93–94
Kittens
    delivery complications of, 2
    Ivermectin and, 44

L
Lacrimal nasal duct, 53
Lameness, 8–9, 59
Lawn chemical poisoning, 96
Lice, 43–45
Lips
    red, 35–36
    swelling, 89
Loose stools, 22–25, 29, 39
Loperamide, 22–24
Lumbar disc rupture, 97–98
Luv My Pet, 7, 74
Luxating patellas, 8–9
Lyme disease, 66–67

M
Maggots, 40–41
Mange, 37–38, 41–42, 43
Marquis, 85–86
Mazola corn oil, 39
Meat-exclusive diets, 25–26
Methanol, 72
Miliary dermatitis, 57
Mites, ear, 1, 43–45, 56–57, 95–96
Morris, Mark M., Jr., 26, 38
Mosquito bite hypersensitivity, 57–58
Motion sickness, 26–28
Mouth, red, 88
Mumps, 90–91
Muscle meats, 25–26

N
Nasal discharge, 51
Nasal vitiligo, 60
Needles, sewing, 80–81
Neutering, 15
Nose
    foreign bodies in, 92
    lack of pigment on, 60
    nasal discharge, 51
Nutrition. *See* Diet

O
Obesity, 6
Omega-3 fatty acids, 58, 76–77
Overfeeding, 6, 11–12

P
Pacific giant salamanders, 63–64
Pale gums, 22, 29
Panacur, 82–84

Parasites, 22–24, 29–33, 43–45, 81–86
   See also Fleas
Parvovirus, 22
Passing gas, 20–21
Patellas, 8–9
Penicillin, 48
Pepcid AC, 34
Pepto-Bismol, 24
Pet foods
   bad breath and, 19–20
   choices of, 11–12
   dull hair coat and, 38
   taurine deficiency and, 67–68
   See also Diet
Pet Poison Helpline, 70–71
Plants, poisonous, 69–70
Plastic feeding bowls, 35–36
Poison control centers, 70–71
Poisoning
   antifreeze, 64–65
   avocado, 73
   chocolate, 66
   emergency helplines, 70–71
   grapes or raisins, 65
   gunpowder, 98
   household hazards, 71–73
   plants, 69–70
   raw egg, 65–66
   salmon, 63–64
   yard chemicals, 96
Ponazuril, 85–86
Praziquantel, 29, 82
ProDen Plaque Off, 20
Proglottids, 8, 82
Pruritus, 8, 77
Puppies
   delivery complications of, 2
   Ivermectin and, 44
   loose stools and, 23
Pyrantel, 29, 82

R
Rabies, 7, 73–74
Raisin toxicity, 65
Rattlesnake bites, 91
Raw eggs, 39, 65–66
Reactions, immunization, 7–8
Red lips, 35–36
Red mange, 37–38, 41–42, 43
Red mouth, 88
Reverse sneeze, 93
Revolution, 40, 96
Rice and cottage cheese diet, 25
Ringworm, 46–47
Robitussin DM, 3, 94
Rocky Mountain spotted fever, 63
Roundworms, 29–30, 43, 82–84
Ruptured intervertebral discs, 97–98

S
Salmon poisoning, 63–64
Salt solution, 65, 66
Scabies, 42, 43–45
Sclera, 54–55
Scooting, 8
Sebaceous gland cysts, 47
Seizures, 10
Self-mutilation, 9–10
Separation anxiety, 98–99
Sewing needles, 80–81
Sewing thread, 81
Shampoos, 60, 72–73
Shedding, 58
Shots. *See* Immunizations
Skin, dry, 60–61
Skin wounds, 42, 48
Skunk treatments, 15–16
Snake bites, 91
Sneezing, 92, 93
Soaps, 72–73
Spastic entropion, 53
Spaying, 15

Stools
    black, 24, 29
    loose, 22–25, 29, 39
Sulfadimethoxine, 30–33, 85
Sulmet, 30–33, 85
Sunstroke, 87–88
Swollen lip, 89
Syrup of ipecac, 65, 66

T
Table scraps, 76
Tapeworms, 8, 29, 81–84
Tartar Shield, 20
Taurine deficiency, 67–68
Teeth
    abscessed tooth, 99
    aging by, 78–79
    bad breath and, 19–20
    yellow tooth syndrome, 77
Terramycin ophthalmic ointment, 54
Tetracycline, 77
Thread, sewing, 81
Tick paralysis, 68–69
Ticks, 63, 66–67, 68–69
Tinactin cream, 47
Toenail bleeding, 11
Toilet water, 64–65
Trachea blockage, 80
Tracheotomy, 5
Traveling with pets, 26–28
Trout, 63–64
Tuf-Foot, 59

U
Umbilical hernias, 95

V
Vaccinations, 7–8, 73–74, 91, 93–94
Vegetable diets, 12
Veterinarian, lying to, 92
Vocal cords, 80
Vomiting
    for attention, 10
    causes of, 34
    induced, 64–65, 66, 71

W
Washington State Poison Center, 71
Weight loss, 6
Whipworms, 29, 82–84
White gums, 22, 29
Windpipe blockage, 80
Worms. *See* Parasites
Wounds, skin, 42, 48

Y
Yard chemical poisoning, 96
Yeast infections, 77
Yellow tooth syndrome, 77

Notes

REED MEMORIAL LIBRARY
1733 Route 6
Carmel, NY 10512
845-225-2439
www.carmellibrary.org